2017 年度
药品检查报告

国家药品监督管理局
年度检查报告系列

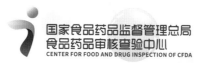

国家食品药品监督管理总局
食品药品审核查验中心
CENTER FOR FOOD AND DRUG INSPECTION OF CFDA

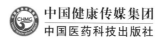

中国健康传媒集团
中国医药科技出版社

图书在版编目（CIP）数据

2017 年度药品检查报告 / 国家食品药品监督管理总局食品药品审核查验中心编写 . — 北京：中国医药科技出版社，2018.8
ISBN 978-7-5214-0385-5

Ⅰ . ① 2… Ⅱ . ① 国… Ⅲ . ① 药品 – 检查 – 调查报告 – 2017 Ⅳ . ① R97

中国版本图书馆 CIP 数据核字（2018）第 188636 号

美术编辑　陈君杞

版式设计　锋尚设计

出版　**中国健康传媒集团** | **中国医药科技出版社**

地址　北京市海淀区文慧园北路甲 22 号

邮编　100082

电话　发行：010-62227427　邮购：010-62236938

网址　www.cmstp.com

规格　787×1092mm　$\frac{1}{16}$

印张　6

字数　88 千字

版次　2018 年 8 月第 1 版

印次　2018 年 8 月第 1 次印刷

印刷　北京瑞禾彩色印刷有限公司

经销　全国各地新华书店

书号　ISBN 978-7-5214-0385-5

定价　48.00 元

编委会

序

2017年度是国家药品监管改革继续深化的重要一年。原国家食品药品监督管理总局落实党中央国务院的要求，以"最严谨的标准、最严格的监管、最严厉的处罚、最严肃的问责"为指导思想，全面加强药品全生命周期监管、落实药品上市许可持有人主体责任，全力推进已上市药品的品质提升，鼓励药品创新。

在原国家食品药品监督管理总局的全面领导下，国家食品药品监督管理总局食品药品审核查验中心聚焦新政策导向，发挥药品检查对监管的有效支撑，严格高效开展药品检查工作。2017年完成了药品注册生产现场检查、仿制药一致性评价检查、药品GMP跟踪检查、飞行检查、进口药品境外生产现场检查、流通检查以及观察检查等各类检查任务。上述药品检查工作的有效开展，在震慑违法违规行为、净化医药行业生态、保证公众用药质量安全方面发挥了重要作用。

本报告包括中英文版，报告的撰写是在原总局药品化妆品监管司、药品化妆品注册管理司的共同指导下完成的，在总结2017年度各类药品检查情况、检查发现的主要问题的基础上，分析了各类检查中发现的药品生产环节质量管理的薄弱环节和潜在质量风险。

国家食品药品监督管理总局食品药品审核查验中心

二〇一八年五月

前　言

2017年原国家食品药品监督管理总局组织开展药品注册生产现场检查、仿制药一致性评价现场检查、药品GMP跟踪检查、飞行检查、进口药品境外生产现场检查、流通检查及国际观察检查共计751项。

2017 年完成各类药品检查任务一览表

检查工作	检查企业数/品种数	派出组数	派出人次
药品注册生产现场检查	52	47	168
仿制药一致性评价检查	12	8	38
药品GMP跟踪检查	428	296	1234
药品飞行检查	57	55	183
进口药品境外生产现场检查	51	41	148
药品流通检查	67	62	202
国际观察检查	84	84	92
合计	751	593	2065

目　录

第一章
药品注册生产现场检查

按照《药品注册管理办法》（国家食品药品监督管理局令第28号）、《药品注册现场核查管理规定》等法规文件的要求，组织开展了药品注册生产现场检查、有因检查工作，同时根据《关于仿制药质量和疗效一致性评价工作有关事项的公告》（国家食品药品监督管理总局公告2017年第100号）开展了仿制药质量和疗效一致性评价的药学、生产现场检查工作。

一、检查基本情况

2017年共有68个检查任务，共派出47个检查组168人次对52个品规进行了现场检查。完成现场检查报告45个，其中通过42个，占比93.3%；不通过3个，占比6.7%。

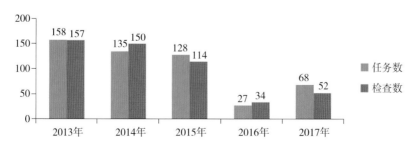

图1-1　近五年药品注册生产现场检查任务数量图

1

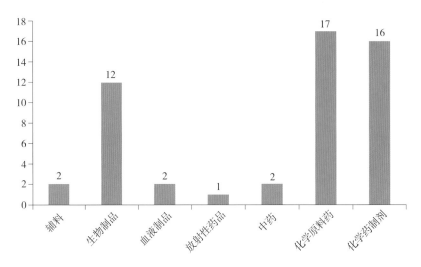

图1-2 2017年注册生产现场检查剂型分布图

二、发现的主要问题

2017年现场检查发现的问题中，申报资料不真实、数据无法溯源等数据可靠性问题已不再突出。这与2017年度注册生产现场检查任务大部分通过了临床试验数据核查、企业在研发过程中对数据可靠性问题普遍提高重视有一定关系。但是，批准上市前药品GMP符合性问题较多，说明企业在药品研发过程中质量管理体系建设比较薄弱，对药品GMP的符合性关注不够。2017年度发现企业存在研发过程中生产质量管理规范执行不足、偏差及超标调查不充分、工艺验证不科学等问题。具体如下：

（一）中试或技术转移过程中药品 GMP 规范执行不足

目前大多数企业已意识到从研发到生产的技术转移需要进行质量管理，但仍存在不足。个别企业仍未将此过程纳入药品GMP体系之中，存在人员职责不清、生产部门对品种工艺知识理解不够、研发部门实施工艺验证未完全遵循药品GMP规定等现象。

（二）偏差、超标结果调查不充分

存在对偏差、超标结果未能及时调查，或者调查不深入、不全面，未能对产生的根本原因进行充分调查。特别是当发现稳定性试验数据偏离趋势的异常数据，未能引起足够重视，未及时开展调查，后期再查找原因变得十分困难。

（三）工艺验证不科学、不充分

部分企业对产品和工艺前期研究不足，对工艺理解不够，药品工艺验证方案设计不科学。工艺验证出现偏差不能按照药品GMP要求进行记录、分析，不能找到根本原因并制定纠正与预防措施。个别企业甚至把连续生产3批合格产品作为判定工艺验证合格的标准。

三、仿制药质量和疗效一致性评价的现场检查工作

2017年11月23日，原国家食品药品监督管理总局启动首批仿制药一致性评价品种的有因检查工作。首批现场检查的7个品种均在完成立卷审查的基础上开展，共派出6个检查组对7个品种的7家研制和生产单位进行了现场检查，涉及9个场地。同时本年度还对5个品种（涉及2家企业）的原研地产化产品进行了现场检查。具体检查品种见下表：

表1-1 原研地产化现场检查品种

序号	检查品种	规格	检查企业
1	尼莫地平片	30mg	拜耳医药保健有限公司
2	阿卡波糖片	50mg；100mg	
3	利培酮片	1mg；2mg	西安杨森制药有限公司
4	盐酸氟桂利嗪胶囊	5mg	
5	多潘立酮片	5mg；10mg	

表 1-2　仿制药一致性评价现场检查品种

序号	检查品种	规格	检查企业
1	阿法骨化醇片	0.25μg；0.5μg	重庆药友制药有限责任公司
2	盐酸阿米替林片	25mg	湖南洞庭药业股份有限公司
3	草酸艾司西酞普兰片	10mg	湖南洞庭药业股份有限公司
4	阿莫西林胶囊	0.25g	浙江康恩贝生物制药有限公司
5	阿托伐他汀钙片	10mg；20mg	北京嘉林药业股份有限公司
6	苯磺酸氨氯地平片	5mg（按$C_{20}H_{25}CIN_{2}O_{5}$计）	江苏黄河药业股份有限公司
7	恩替卡韦分散片	0.5mg	江西青峰药业有限公司

第二章
药品 GMP 跟踪检查

2017年药品GMP跟踪检查遵循"以风险为基础，以品种为主线"的原则，采取"双随机""回头看"等多种方式，在总结过去两年跟踪检查经验的基础上，综合分析国家抽验、不良反应监测等风险信号制定国家药品检查计划，并按计划开展药品GMP跟踪检查。

一、检查基本情况

根据《2017年国家药品检查计划》，2017年计划对315家风险较高的企业和150家"双随机"抽取的企业开展跟踪检查。其中有37家企业因未通过药品GMP认证、药品GMP证书被收回、无相应药品批准文号等原因不具备现场检查条件。全年共完成药品GMP跟踪检查428家（478家次），较2016年同比增长234%。对于跟踪检查发现问题的企业都已依法依规进行了处理。

表 2-1　检查派组情况

检查总数（家次）	检查组数	检查员人次
428	296	1234

表 2-2　检查分布情况

类别		检查数量（家次）
风险较高的企业	上次跟踪检查结论为不通过、有严重缺陷或主要缺陷超过3项、发过告诫信的企业，国外药品监管机构检查发现问题的企业，注册生产现场检查发现有必要进行跟踪检查的企业，2015年飞行检查原国家食品药品监督管理总局公告的企业等	114
	疫苗类生物制品生产企业	39
	血液制品生产企业	26
	2016年国家抽验不合格及抽验发现问题较多	27
	不良反应监测发现ADR或预警事件	8
	专项检查品种	123
双随机检查企业	麻醉药品、精神药品和药品类易制毒类生产企业	15
	中药材及饮片	48
	2016年省认证企业	30
	中药提取物	15
	生化药	17
	中药注射剂	16
合计	单位：家次	478
	单位：家	428

　　2017年药品GMP跟踪检查结论为不符合的企业共37家，占8.6%，发告诫信的企业108家，占25%。具体分布情况如下：

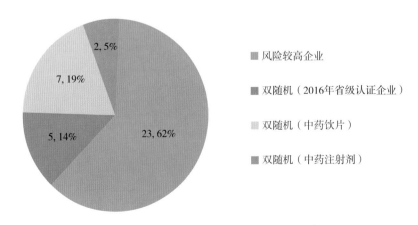

图2-1　2017年跟踪检查不符合企业分布情况

图注：检查不符合的原因包括严重违反药品GMP、涉嫌违法、产品质量不稳定等多种因素，不同原因导致不符合的处理措施存在不同

二、发现的主要问题

（一）总体情况

428家药品生产企业的检查发现药品GMP缺陷4339项，其中涉及药品GMP正文部分的缺陷共3512项，涉及计算机化系统附录的缺陷224项，涉及无菌药品附录的缺陷200项，涉及中药饮片的缺陷116项。

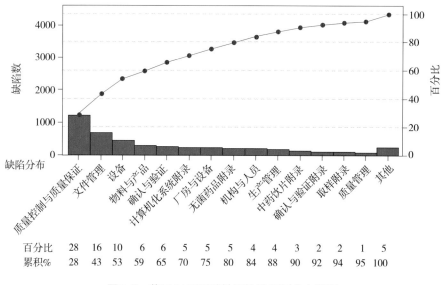

图2-2　药品GMP跟踪检查缺陷项目分布情况

如图2-2所示，在质量控制与质量保证部分发现的缺陷最多，共1205条，占全部缺陷的28%；其次是文件管理，占比16%；再次是设备，占比10%。

对提出缺陷的条款进行分析，频次超过20次的条款进行统计如图2-3：

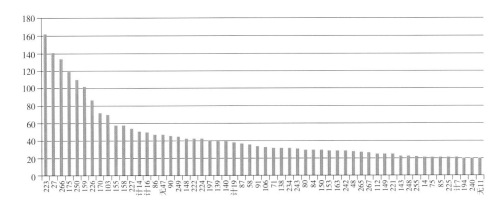

图2-3 药品GMP跟踪检查不符合条款分布情况

图注："计"表示计算机化系统附录，"无"表示无菌药品附录

缺陷不符合最多的条款是第223条（药品检验），其次是第27条（人员培训），排第三位的是第266条（产品质量回顾分析），第四位的是第175条（批生产记录），第五位的是第250条（偏差调查及预防措施）。

整体上看，当前我国药品生产企业存在的问题主要集中于以下几个方面：质量控制与质量保证、文件管理、设备、物料与产品、确认与验证、计算机化系统附录、厂房与设施、无菌药品附录、机构与人员、生产管理、中药饮片附录、确认与验证附录、取样附录及质量管理等。上述缺陷占全部缺陷的95%，其中前八项占比80%。常见的一些问题包括：

（1）药品检验操作不符合要求，部分分析方法未经确认，检验用对照品、标准物质和菌种管理不规范，相关检验记录管控不足，记录信息不全，追溯性差。

（2）培训管理不符合要求，培训计划和培训方案针对性不强，部分人员培训效果较差，GMP相关工作内容未进行培训。

（3）产品质量回顾规定不合理，回顾内容未涵盖产品关键信息，回顾数据与实际情况不一致，回顾发现的异常情况未采取相应措施。

（4）批记录信息不完整，可追溯性差，存在记录不规范、不及时等情况。

（5）偏差管理系统不能有效运行，一些偏差未开展偏差调查，部分偏差调查不充分。

（6）工艺规程中缺少部分操作的描述或描述不清晰，部分信息变更后未及时修订工艺规程。

（7）物料管理不规范，相关标识、记录信息不完整，可追溯性差，储存环境不符合要求。

（8）计算机化系统附录方面，主要是权限设置不合理，电子数据管理存在不足，审计追踪功能不完善等问题。

（9）无菌药品附录方面，在培养基模拟灌装试验和洁净区监测方面的问题比较集中，包括培养基模拟灌装试验不科学、洁净区监控记录未纳入批生产记录中审核等。

通过对检查不符合的企业缺陷进行分析，导致不符合的主要问题包括：

（1）存在严重数据可靠性问题，包括修改系统时间后检测、关键数据无法溯源，原始记录、原始图谱、原始数据及计算过程缺失，检验原始记录内容不一致，恶意修改积分参数，套用图谱，生产和检验记录管理混乱，提前填写记录，未对分析仪器的计算机系统进行权限管理和有效控制等。

（2）质量管理体系不能有效运行，存在系统性问题。如人员资质和数量与生产要求不匹配，未对偏差、超标结果进行有效识别、调查，变更未执行变更控制程序等。

（3）物料质量控制不符合要求。如未按照《中国药典》（2015年版）进行有效红外鉴别，物料账物不符等。

（4）未经注册批准擅自在处方中增加辅料，擅自修改关键工艺参数后生产。

（5）违法外购中药饮片进行分包装。

（6）产品质量不可控。

（7）实际生产工艺与注册申报工艺不一致。

（二）疫苗类生物制品生产企业检查情况

2017年对持有药品GMP证书的疫苗生产企业进行了100%覆盖检查，除1家企业因搬迁停产及计划注销GMP证书未实施检查外，对剩余39家企业均进行了检查。

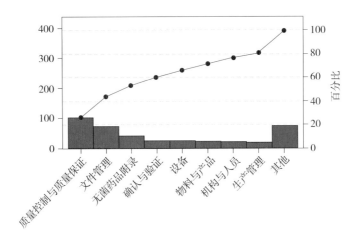

图2-4　疫苗生产企业缺陷分布图

疫苗生产企业检查缺陷主要集中在质量控制与质量保证、文件管理、无菌药品附录、确认与验证、设备、物料与产品、机构与人员、生产管理部分。检查中发现的比较突出问题如下：

（1）在工艺验证的实施方面，存在没有确定产品的关键质量属性、关键工艺参数及范围等问题。

（2）无菌工艺模拟试验方面没考虑最差条件，起始点没有从无菌操作的第一步开始模拟。

（3）一些企业使用一瓶原液用于多批成品的配制，多次开瓶存在污染风险。

（4）使用佐剂的质量标准不能反映佐剂的性能，也未对佐剂配制工艺、性能确认。

（5）中间产品的配制和分装的均一性验证存在取样量不足的情况。

（6）一些企业因产品生产季节性，存在招聘临时人员从事质量控制工作的情况。

（7）一些企业未严格执行《中国药典》（2015年版）规定，如减毒活疫苗主种子未进行全基因测序。

（8）一些企业年度质量回顾内容不全，没有将批签发不合格批次、撤检批次列入统计的情况。

（三）血液制品生产企业检查情况

2017年对持有药品GMP证书的血液制品生产企业进行了100%覆盖检查，除1家因药品GMP证书被回收未实施检查外，其余26家血液制品生产企业均进行了跟踪检查。

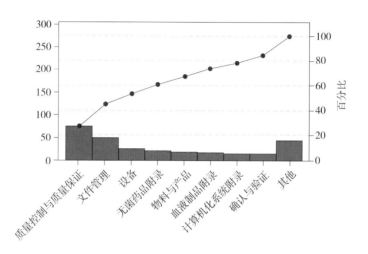

图2-5　血液制品生产企业缺陷分布图

血液制品生产企业缺陷主要集中在质量控制与质量保证、文件管理、设备、无菌药品附录、物料与产品、血液制品附录、计算机化系统附录、确认与验证部分。检查中发现的比较突出问题如下：

（1）部分企业在产品效期内铝离子含量有上升的趋势，企业未及时启动相关调查或调查不彻底。

（2）部分企业存在乙醇回收情况，相关研究不足。

（3）年度质量回顾报告未能指导后续改进、提升工作。

（四）四类专项产品检查情况

按照2017年检查计划，对桔丙酯系列产品、胞磷胆碱钠原料药、长春西汀注射剂和丹参注射剂等四类产品进行了跟踪检查，检查共发现缺陷1243项，其中桔丙酯系列产品检查发现缺陷365项（包括严重缺陷4项、主要缺陷31项、一般缺陷330项），胞磷胆碱钠检查发现缺陷59项（包括主要缺陷6项、一般缺陷53项），丹参注射剂检查发现缺陷486项（包括主要缺陷38项、一般缺陷448项），长春西汀注射剂检查发现缺陷333项（包括主要缺陷26项、一般缺陷307项）具体分布如下：

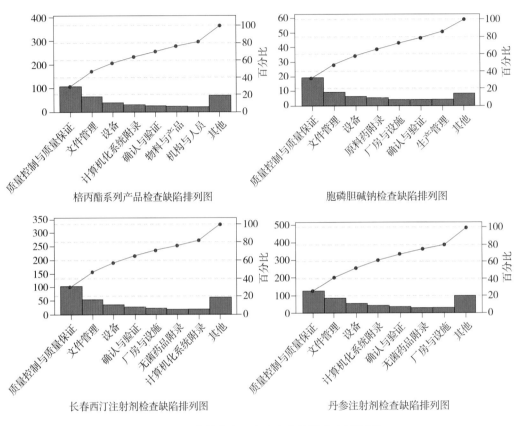

图2-6　四类特定产品生产企业缺陷分布排列图

上述四类产品缺陷分布情况基本与整体检查缺陷分布情况一致。检查过程中针对一些企业对应产品在近期不生产的情况，检查组基于风险原则选择较高风险的产品进行检查。检查发现企业在偏差处理、变更控制、验证科学性、设备维护、记录完整性、数据管理规范性、年度产品质量回顾等方面的问题较突出。其中严重缺陷包括质量管理体系存在系统性问题、关键物料质量控制不符合要求、擅自改变处方后生产、存在较大污染与交叉污染的风险等。

（五）双随机检查情况

2017年共对141家企业开展了双随机检查，共发现缺陷1283项，其中严重缺陷8项，主要缺陷122项，一般缺陷1153项。具体分布如下：

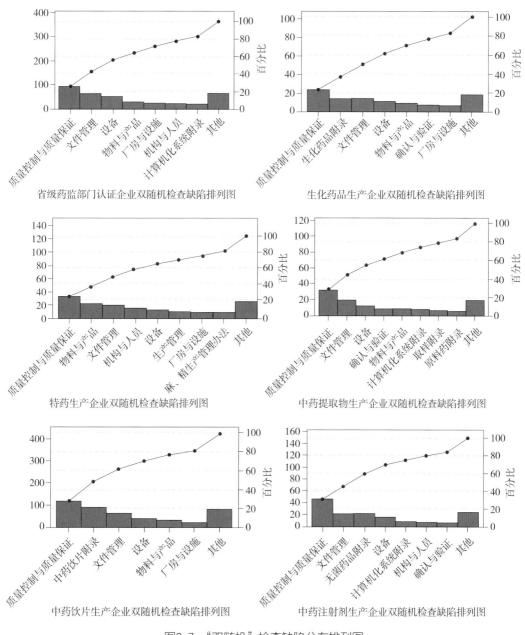

省级药监部门认证企业双随机检查缺陷排列图

生化药品生产企业双随机检查缺陷排列图

特药生产企业双随机检查缺陷排列图

中药提取物生产企业双随机检查缺陷排列图

中药饮片生产企业双随机检查缺陷排列图

中药注射剂生产企业双随机检查缺陷排列图

图2-7　"双随机"检查缺陷分布排列图

　　整体上看，质量控制与质量保证部分的缺陷在各类生产企业的检查缺陷项中均排第一位。根据生产企业类型的不同，缺陷不符合情况存在一定的差异。省级药监部门认证企业、中药提取物生产企业和中药注射剂生产企业双随机检查的缺陷分布情况基本与整体缺陷分布情况一致。生化药品生产企业检查中，不符合生化药品附录的缺陷排第二位，主要是在供应链管理和避免交叉污染的措施方面存在不足。麻醉药品、精神药品和药品类易制毒类生产企业检查发现存在不符合《麻醉药品和精神药品生产管理办法》的情况，主要问题集中在特殊药品管控方面，包括检验剩余样品、生产过程不合格品的控制等。中药饮片生产企业检查发现的不符合条款中，居第二位的是中药饮片附录，主要问题包括购入药材检验、药材留样、药材养护、人员素质和操作规范性等方面。

第三章
药品飞行检查

按照《药品医疗器械飞行检查办法》规定，2017年原国家食品药品监督管理总局对药品生产企业开展了飞行检查及相关延伸检查。

一、检查基本情况

2017年共开展药品GMP飞行检查57家次。涉及吉林、四川、福建等21个省（市），包括5家生物制品生产企业（含血液制品）、14家普通化学药品生产企业、28家中药制剂生产企业、7家中药饮片生产企业和3家中药提取物生产企业。其中占比最高的是中药制剂生产企业，占全部飞行检查工作的49%。中药饮片占比约12%，普通化学药品占比约25%，生物制品占比约9%。

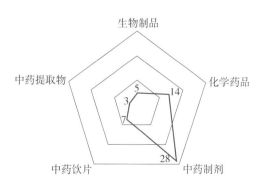

图3-1　药品飞行检查剂型分布情况

全年飞行检查发现存在问题的共有39家企业，占比约68%，其中有27家问题严重的企业要求省局收回GMP证书或立案查处。

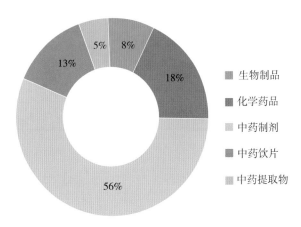

图3-2　药品飞行检查发现严重问题的品种分布情况

2017年飞行检查对中药类生产企业的检查较为集中，针对中药制剂、中药饮片、中药提取物生产企业共派出30个检查组129人次对38家企业进行了飞行检查。其中全国评价性抽验探索性研究发现问题的有16家企业，信访举报的有12家企业，针对检查发现问题开展延伸检查的有8家企业，经研判发现风险较高的企业2家。38家中药类生产企业的飞行检查中共有29家企业不符合相关要求，其中21家企业被收回药品GMP证书，符合要求的共有7家企业，2家企业已无相关生产资质。

二、发现的主要问题

（一）中药类企业发现的主要问题

1. 中成药生产企业

（1）不按处方标准投料。

检查发现该类违法违规的中成药生产企业只要求最终产品能够满足法定的质量控制标准，不考虑药品的安全性、有效性和患者的权益，主观故意不按处方标准投料生产。比如：

- 湖北康源药业有限公司，其一批鹿角胶的生产投料配方是熬骆驼皮时的上层白沫，再添加鹿皮熬制的胶，生产处方中未见鹿角。一批龟甲胶的生产投料配方是以单一杂皮胶和多种杂皮胶为主，再添加部分不合格胶，最后加入约5%的龟甲胶。

- 吉林省鑫辉药业有限公司生产藿香正气水，437批藿香正气水甘草浸膏的实际投料量只是标准投料量的18%，广藿香油的实际投料量仅是标准投料量的28%。

（2）违背法定制法，擅自改变工艺。

2017年飞行检查发现的该类问题集中体现在企业为了降低生产成本或使用不合格原药材投料将处方中部分应提取的中药材不按标准提取，而是粉碎后直接投料。问题举例如下：

- 炎可宁片的处方由五味药材组成，其中黄柏药材需单独处理——水煎煮三次，合并浓缩后加乙醇静置、滤过，回收乙醇，浓缩。企业均出于降低原药材成本、降低工艺生产成本的原因，将黄柏药材直接粉碎进入制剂工序投料，飞行检查发现三家企业存在上述问题。

- 清热解毒片在《中国药典》（2010版）第三增补本中，增加了栀子苷含量检测指标（≥0.6mg/片）。个别企业因生产投料的栀子药材不合格，故在正常生产外每批产品制剂工序还要单独添加栀子药材原粉，以保证最终产品检验栀子苷含量检测符合要求。

（3）为应对监督检查，编造相关记录文件。

2017年的飞行检查发现多家企业存在两套甚至三套物料账、物料出入库记录和生产批记录的情况。

- 湖北康源药业有限公司内部有三套账，真实的一套供企业内部使用，第二套是为应对抽检不合格预减轻处罚而设立的"低收率"账目，第三套是为应对市场反馈价格偏低而设立的"高收率"账目。

- 安徽济人药业有限公司存在两套物料账和批生产记录，一套是为了应对监督检查，其处方和生产工艺与注册标准完全一致，另一套是实际的批生产记录，与注册标准不一致。

2．中药饮片生产企业

2017年，对中药饮片的飞行检查主要针对外购中药饮片直接进行分装、销售，购进中药材或炮制后的产品不按标准进行检验，以及染色、增重等问题。检查发现为应对监督检查，一些企业存在编造批生产记录和批检验记录的行为。

（1）外购饮片直接分装、销售。

- 亳州市豪门中药饮片有限公司中药饮片成品库中所有的饮片未建立物料库卡，保管员仅销售后建立了成品出入库分类账。西红花产品留样记录显示2016年10月以来企业共生产了3批西红花（161101、161201、170201），但企业无法提供3批产品的批生产记录。

- 安国路路通中药饮片有限公司熟地黄、黄精、酒苁蓉、酒萸肉、酒女贞子、酒大黄的生产需使用黄酒作为辅料，上述品种2016年以来均有正常生产，但企业生产用黄酒的《2017年辅料总账与分类明细账》与现场实物存在严重不符，且无法供货单位销售黄酒的增值税专用发票。

- 武山县医药公司所属的中药饮片生产企业，在《药品生产许可证》有效期到期后停止生产，并将厂房出让。但该企业相关人员继续直接采购中药饮片直接分装，套用企业停产前的生产批号，通过其上级医药公司进行销售。

（2）未按照标准对购入或销售的中药材、中药饮片进行全检。

- 不能提供对应药材检测设备使用登记记录。

- 缺少药材检验用对照品、毛细管柱，无对应项目检测能力，但仍出具全检报告。

（3）批生产记录不真实。

- 不能提供主要生产设备的使用日志，特定药材批生产记录显示用量与领料单显示用量相差5倍，部分生产用辅料批生产记录用量前后不一致。

- 批生产记录中员工签名不真实。

3．中药提取物的生产备案

2017年选取了两家低价销售的藿香正气水生产企业进行飞行检查，同时延伸至三家甘草浸膏、广藿香油的中药提取物生产厂进行检查。发现企业还是有不同形式的违反《食品药品监管总局关于加强中药生产中提取和提取物监督管理的通知》（食药监药化监〔2014〕135号）的情况。具体问题如下：

- 四川禾邦旭东制药有限公司在2016年1月26日按规定对甘草浸膏、广藿香油进行外购提取物备案的同时，自2016年2月起即开始了私自进行甘草浸膏和广藿香油的提取。该企业还恶意编制其他中药提取物生产企业的票据，私刻其他中药提取物生产企业的出库专用章，编造相关的物料台账、批生产记录以应对监督检查。

- 广东同德药业有限公司尽管通过省食品药品监督管理局备案，但其不具备生产广藿香油的主要生产设备，而是在药材产地收购粗油，对不合格的广藿香油增加一道精制工序，经本企业中药提取车间再精制后进行销售。

（二）化学药品生产企业发现的主要问题

2017年共对14家普通化学药品生产企业进行了飞行检查，发现其中有7家企业存在问题。主要问题集中在以下几个方面：

1．违反注册批准工艺生产

违法外购原料粗品生产本公司原料药。企业不能提供能够追溯原料药生产的起始物料来源记录，不能提供追溯药品生产、质量管理过程的相关记录。原料药无任何物料、生产、检验记录即放行销售，关键人员未履行职责。

2．检测原始数据无法溯源，数据可靠性存在严重问题

随意开启、删除审计追踪日志。设备所用电脑系统时间可以修改，且系统日志中出现2016、2017年修改系统时间的记录；更改系统时间后进行有关物质检测。

部分超标调查处理不彻底，如超标结果调查描述到检验及取样过程无异常，但仍重新取样复检合格后放行。

3．采用不合格原料生产药品

使用不符合《中国药典》（2015年版）标准的原料药生产片剂并上市销售；伪造、更换原料药生产企业标签，伪造原料药生产企业检验报告书；更换检验样品和留样样品，部分原料药进厂检验结果不真实；企业关键管理人员不能依法依规履职尽责，直接参与实施违法行为。

（三）生物制品生产企业发现的主要问题

2017年共对5家生物制品生产企业进行了飞行检查，发现其中有3家企业存

在问题。主要问题集中在以下几个方面：

1. 过程控制数据或产品结果数据不真实

广州丹霞生物制药有限公司用于申报生产注册的9个批次的人血白蛋白长期稳定性考察3个月、6个月、加速试验6个月大部分铝离子实际检测结果高于《中国药典》规定的200μg/L的标准。该生物制品上市后持续稳定性考察铝离子检测结果与报告不一致，实际检测结果不符合标准，企业存在修改样品名、删除检测记录重新检测等问题。

杭州普济医药技术开发有限公司伪造中间品和成品检测数据、猪全血分离的血浆微生物限度检测数据、猪血冷藏车运输温度记录、纯化水系统验证微生物限度检测数据、培养基模拟灌装试验培养室温度监测数据、洁净区空气监测数据、上市批次的冻干工艺批生产记录等，并掩盖不合格产品真实原因的有关数据、篡改QC实验室计算机系统时间等。

2. 实际生产工艺与产品注册工艺不一致

产品实际生产工艺催化剂活化工序存在反复活化操作的行为与注册批准工艺不一致。

3. 使用不符合质量标准的原材料、中间体及半成品进行投料

采用微生物标准不合格的血浆进行试验批投料生产；采用乙醇残留量、细菌内毒素、凝固活力、微生物限度、纯度、氯化钡残留量不合格的中间体和pH值、蛋白浓度、酶活力不合格的半成品进行投料。

4. 生产工艺及批量变更未进行相关研究

催化剂精制工序由6000分子量的超滤膜变更为10000分子量的超滤膜包，无验证数据支持此变更；催化剂超滤工序中重复超滤，未进行相关验证研究；主体胶纯化及精制工序变更滤芯组合，由滤芯变更为滤饼，除菌过滤工序材质由PVDF变更为PES，未进行相关验证研究或验证数据不充分；溶解液批量由2万瓶变更至4万瓶，未进行相关验证研究。

5. 铝佐剂质量控制问题

未进行氢氧化铝佐剂对抗原吸附效果的检测，未开展佐剂氢氧化铝对产品质量影响的研究。氢氧化铝作为重要的辅料（佐剂）没有进行有效的质量控制。

第四章
进口药品境外生产现场检查

一、检查基本情况

2017年原国家食品药品监督管理总局共派出41个检查组148名检查员完成了51个品种的进口药品境外生产现场检查任务。

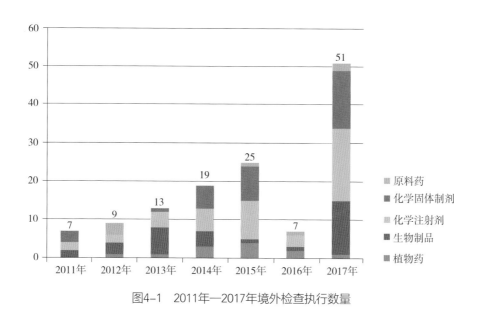

图4-1　2011年—2017年境外检查执行数量

2017年境外检查品种剂型较多，其中加大了对化学药品制剂延伸检查力度。全年任务中包括化学药品36个，含注射剂、固体制剂、粉雾剂、原料药等，疫苗、血液制品、治疗用生物制品14个，植物药1个。全年境外检查药品包括申报生产、再注册、补充申请阶段及正常进口销售的产品。主要集中在欧洲、北美地区，对印度等国家的检查数量呈增长趋势。

二、发现的主要问题

对51个开展现场检查的品种中，9个品种现场检查结论为不符合药品GMP要求或不通过，根据产品处于的不同阶段（上市前审评或已上市），都已经分别进行了处理。8个未开展现场检查的品种中，6个品种企业已主动采取风险控制措施，其余的列入下年度检查计划中。

检查共发现缺陷项665项，其中严重缺陷27项，主要缺陷140项。问题主要集中在质量控制与质量保证、文件管理、无菌药品管理等方面。严重缺陷主要包括生产工艺不一致、重大变更未及时向我国申报，注册申报资料存在真实性问题，生产厂房设施、设备和生产操作行为等不能有效降低产品污染或混淆的风险，不能对不合格产品进行有效控制等方面。

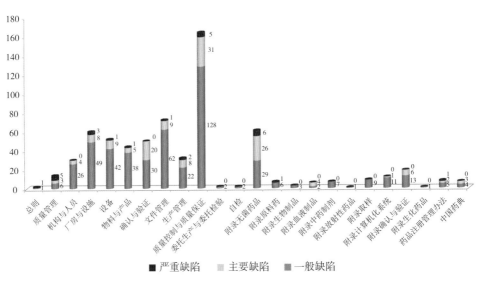

图4-2　2017年境外检查缺陷分布情况

根据出现缺陷频次统计，质量控制与质量保证部分发现缺陷最多，共164项（占比24.7%）；其次是文件管理部分，发现缺陷72项（占比10.8%），无菌药品附录部分发现缺陷61项（占比9.2%）。常见问题包括：

（1）偏差管理系统不能有效运行，一些偏差未开展调查，部分偏差调查不充分。

（2）药品检验取样操作和记录不符合要求；未对纯化水生产过程数据进行监控和验证；检验数据、环境监测数据采用不便于趋势分析的方法保存。

（3）批生产记录记录信息不足，如缺少灌装后已灭菌剩余胶塞和铝盖的数量和去向。

（4）年度回顾报告不完整，如没有对趋势分析规定纠偏限、警戒限。

（5）生产工艺规程内容制定不完整，如：缺少部分工艺参数（乳化温度、剪切速度等、隧道灭菌烘箱停留的最长时限、氮气压力等）规定。

（6）无菌药品附录中培养基模拟灌装验证不科学的问题较集中，如验证频次不合理、最差条件未考虑生产线最多允许人数、储罐灭菌后放置时间等。

2017年境外检查中，企业出现检查不通过的主要问题包括：

（1）实际生产工艺、生产场地、检验项目等与注册申报不一致，或有重大变更等情况未向我国进行申报即已执行。如注射剂油相配制过程中，实际过滤方式、滤材与注册申报资料不一致；放行出口中国的产品未按进口注册标准进行有关物质检验及含量均匀度的测定；改变工艺处方；实际生产厂、生产地址与进口药品注册证标示的生产厂和生产地址不符等。

（2）存在严重数据可靠性问题。如多批次释放度检测图谱使用粘贴信息纸条进行复印伪造的材料作为提交注册审评的资料；现场检查无法提供原始检验记录；处方筛选样品试制批号与有关中间品、成品检验的批号不一致，同一批次样品试制记录、颗粒含量测定、释放度测定（成品）、含量测定（素片）批号不一致等。

（3）生产厂房设施、设备和生产操作行为等不能有效降低产品污染或混淆的风险。如注射水针配置灌装生产线与粉针制剂生产线（该生产线有激素类产品）位于同一车间，共用空气净化系统，企业未进行风险评估也未能采取有效防护措施以避免激素类产品对其他产品的污染；灌装操作人员需手工将胶塞压进铝盖，再将其放置于已灌装的三腔袋相应腔口；厂区内多处污水、垃圾；一般生产区防蚊虫措施不力，生产厂区常年高温（最高45℃），无降温措施，门窗不能密闭；纱窗多处破损，生产现场多处发现蚊虫；多处敞口投料或转料操作，无局部保护等。

（4）产品质量不可控制。在一项因进口检验细菌内毒素项目不合格启动的现场检查中发现企业重新检测该项目仍不符合规定未进行超标结果调查，未对产品及其所用原料药前后生产的相关批次进行风险评估；未按《中国药典》进行全检等。

第五章
药品流通检查

为进一步加强药品流通环节质量监管，规范药品经营秩序，2017年原国家食品药品监督管理总局组织了对药品批发企业的跟踪检查和对零售药店的检查。

一、检查基本情况

（一）任务概况

按照《2017年药品GSP跟踪检查计划》，全年共组织完成药品批发企业跟踪检查55家，涵盖广东、四川、湖北等20个省（自治区，直辖市）。为部署城乡接合部和农村地区药店诊所药品质量安全集中整治，还组织对辽宁、湖南、贵州3省12家零售药店进行了飞行检查。与2016年检查任务相比，本年度检查任务增加34%，检查情况如下。

表 5-1 2016、2017 年度药品流通检查任务量

年度	检查企业数（家）	派出人数（人次）
2016	50	77
2017	67	202
总计	117	206

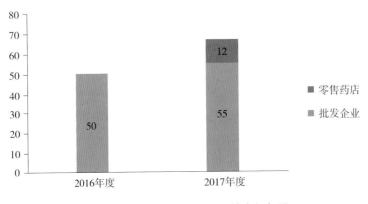

图5-1 2016、2017药品流通检查任务量

（二）检查原则及检查范围

按照风险管控原则，本年度药品流通跟踪检查选择经营品种安全风险高、品种储存条件要求高、有国家药品抽检不合格、有过被投诉举报的药品批发企业进行跟踪检查，检查采取"双随机"方式，从全国药品批发企业中按不同类型随机抽取55家批发企业，从城乡接合部和农村地区药店中抽取12家零售药店进行了检查，见表5-2。

表 5-2 药品 GSP 检查范围

类别	企业数（家）
经营麻醉药品和精神药品（含复方制剂）	15
经营范围含生物制品、冷链药品	15
新开办企业	15
国家药品抽检不合格	5
被投诉举报	5
城乡接合部和农村地区零售药店	12
共计	67

（三）检查结果

依据《药品经营质量管理规范现场检查指导原则》，29家经营企业严重违反《药品经营质量管理规范》，结果判定为检查不通过。

（1）经营麻醉药品和精神药品（含复方制剂）的批发企业：3家检查不通过，占检查企业数15家的20%。

（2）经营范围含生物制品、冷链药品的批发企业：1家处于歇业状态，检查无结论，6家检查不通过，占检查企业数15家的40%。

（3）新开办批发企业：5家检查不通过，占检查企业数15家的33.3%。

（4）有国家药品抽检不合格的批发企业：2家检查不通过，占检查企业数5家的40%。

（5）有过投诉举报的批发企业：3家（其中1家处于GSP认证公示期间）检查不通过，占检查企业数5家的60%。

（6）城乡接合部和农村地区零售药店：10家检查不通过，占检查企业数12家的83.3%。

综上，药品批发企业跟踪检查不通过企业19家，不通过率34.5%。城乡接合部和农村地区零售药店飞行检查不通过企业10家，不通过率83.3%。与2016年检查情况对比，批发企业不通过率出现明显下降。对于检查不通过的企业，都已依法依规进行了处理。

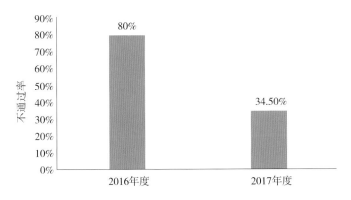

图5-2　2016、2017年药品批发企业检查不通过率

二、发现的主要问题

（一）药品批发企业检查情况

本年度对药品批发企业的跟踪检查共发现缺陷436项，其中严重缺陷58项，主要缺陷330项，一般缺陷48项。各类型缺陷分布情况见下图：

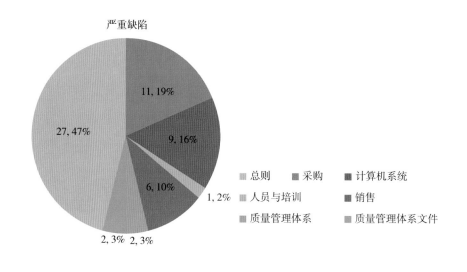

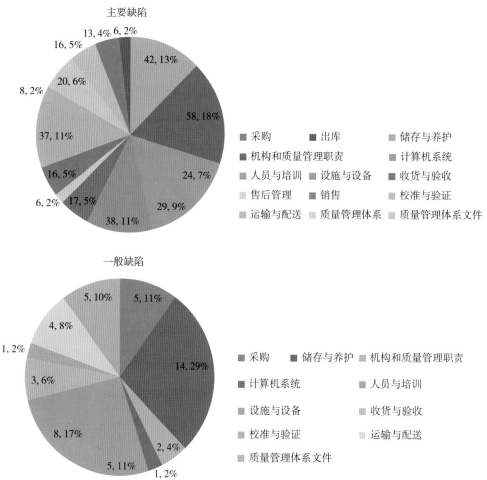

图5-3 药品批发企业缺陷分布

药品批发企业严重缺陷主要分布在总则、采购、计算机系统、销售等方面。药品批发企业主要缺陷主要分布在机构和质量管理职责、储存与养护、设施与设备、校准与验证等方面。药品批发企业一般缺陷主要分布在储存与养护、设施与设备、采购、人员与培训等方面。

1. 经营麻醉药品和精神药品（含复方制剂）的批发企业检查情况

该类15家企业检查共存在缺陷115项，其中严重缺陷10项，分布在总则、计算机系统、质量管理体系，占全部缺陷的8.7%，主要缺陷90项，一般缺陷15项。

检查发现的缺陷较多存在于机构和质量管理职责、校准与验证、设施与设备、采购、计算机系统、人员与培训等方面。现场检查时，检查组除对企业经营符合GSP情况进行检查外，还对其特殊管理药品经营情况进行了针对性检查，必要时根据情况对下游进行了延伸检查。检查发现，大部分企业特药经营情况较好，主要存在一些个别问题，如：邮寄麻醉药品和精神药品未办理准予邮寄证明；不能提供特殊药品运输证明等。

2. 经营范围含生物制品、冷链药品的批发企业检查情况

该类15家企业检查共存在缺陷115项，其中严重缺陷14项，分布在总则、计算机系统、采购，占全部缺陷的12.2%，主要缺陷94项，一般缺陷7项。

检查发现的缺陷较多存在于机构和质量管理职责、设施与设备、校准与验证、储存与养护、计算机系统、人员与培训等方面。由于此类企业经营冷藏、冷冻药品，检查组特别关注其冷链情况。企业存在共性问题包括：冷藏设施设备不符合要求；验证不符合规定；从事冷藏药品储存、运输人员操作培训不到位；部分温湿度记录缺失；冷库温湿度超标后不能及时报警和发送短信；冷藏药品运送过程未能记录温度数据等。

3. 新开办批发企业检查情况

该类15家企业检查共存在缺陷132项，其中严重缺陷21项，分布在总则、采购、销售，占全部缺陷的15.9%，主要缺陷95项，一般缺陷16项。

检查发现的缺陷较多存在于储存与养护、设施与设备、机构和质量管理职责、人员与培训、采购等方面。新开办企业存在问题较前两类企业有所增加，严重缺陷比例上升，如深泽县医药药材公司永济批发部存在缺陷30项，其中严重缺陷9项，违反《关于整治药品流通领域违法经营行为的公告》（国家食品药品监督管理总局公告2016年第94号，以下简称94号公告）1～10项；重庆恩康医药有限公司存在缺陷9项，其中严重缺陷4项，违反94号公告第1、4、5、10项。新开办批发企业存在共性问题包括：未按包装标示的温度要求储存药品；未对库房温湿度进行有效监测、调控；堆垛不符合要求；药品、非药品未分开存放；温湿度监控数据不能合理备份；质量管理人员兼职或未在岗等。

4. 国家药品抽检不合格的批发企业检查情况

该类5家企业检查共存在缺陷36项，其中严重缺陷4项，分布在总则、采购、计算机系统，占全部缺陷的11.1%，主要缺陷29项，一般缺陷3项。

检查发现的缺陷较多存在于机构和质量管理职责、储存与养护、设施与设备等方面。企业存在共性问题包括：设置岗位未制定岗位职责；药品质量档案填写内容不全；质量管理部门验收管理不到位；部分岗位未分配计算机系统操作权限；不同药品混品种码放；温湿度记录备份不符合要求；温湿度监测设施设备不符合规范要求等。

5. 被投诉举报的批发企业检查情况

该类5家企业检查共存在缺陷38项，其中严重缺陷9项，分布于总则、质量管理体系文件、计算机系统、销售，占全部缺陷的23.7%，主要缺陷22项，一般缺陷7项。

检查发现的缺陷较多存在于储存与养护、总则、机构和质量管理职责等。此类企业严重缺陷比其他企业均高，且主要存在于总则部分。企业存在共性问题包括：涉嫌违法经营行为；存在虚假、欺骗行为；药品流向，温湿度监测数据、计算机系统数据等无法追溯；未按要求温度储存药品；未对温湿度进行有效监控；企业存在外部人员兼职行为；质量负责人未独立履行职责等。

（二）城乡接合部和农村地区零售药店检查情况

该类12家企业检查共存在缺陷91项，其中严重缺陷31项，分布于总则、采购与验收，占全部缺陷的34.1%，主要缺陷50项，一般缺陷10项。

检查发现的缺陷较多存在于陈列与储存、采购与验收、总则等方面。城乡接合部和农村地区零售药店检查不通过率为83.3%，严重缺陷比例最高。企业存在共性问题包括：未能提供购进药品的随货同行单、发票，不能追溯该药品的来源；中药饮片未标识生产企业、无外包装、无产地、无生产批号；超范围经营药品、涉嫌从非法渠道购进药品；处方药与非处方药未分区陈列、处方药开架销售；违规销售米非司酮片；伪造处方、计算机系统自动生成处方等。

综上，94号公告发布以来，各级药品监管部门对药品流通企业开展了多轮的飞行检查及跟踪检查（飞行检查形式），严厉打击流通领域违法违规行为，药品经营秩序有所改善。2016年，原国家食品药品监督管理总局对50家药品批发企业进行的飞行检查，其中38家存在严重缺陷，检查通过率仅为24%。本年度对55家批发企业进行检查，其中19家存在严重缺陷，检查通过率65.5%，企业经营行为日趋规范。随着检查力度不断加大，药品流通行业合规意识在逐步增强，违法违规现象逐渐减少。检查促进了行业良性竞争和健康有序发展，为公众用药安全提供有力保障。

第六章
国外机构 GMP 观察检查

根据国外药品监管及检查机构的通知，原国家食品药品监督管理总局对国外药品监管及检查机构对我国药品生产企业的现场检查进行了观察，以掌握我国药品生产企业产品出口及生产质量管理情况，掌握主要国际组织和国外药品监管机构检查情况，评估分析风险信号、为药品检查工作提供参考。

一、检查基本情况

2017年共组织完成国外观察检查84次，涉及企业81家，涵盖浙江、广东等23个省（市、区），其中浙江、广东、北京、河北、江苏、山东占60%，与上年度相比基本一致。

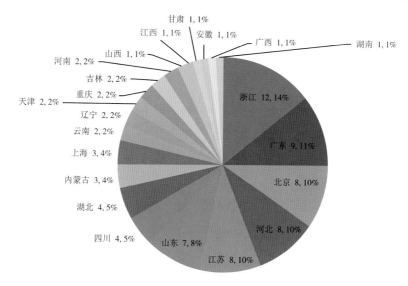

图6-1　2017年国外药品检查观察各省（市）分布情况

2017年检查观察涉及的检查机构包括美国食品药品管理局（US FDA）、世界卫生组织（WHO）、欧洲药品质量理事会（EDQM）、德国汉堡健康及消费者保护部（BGV）、巴西卫生监督局（ANVISA）、印度药物管制总局（DCGI）、英国药品与健康产品管理局（MHRA）、意大利药品管理局（AIFA）、泰国食品药品管理局、荷兰健康监察局（IGZ）、联合国儿童基金会（UNICEF）、欧洲药品管理局（EMA）、坦桑尼亚食品药品监督管理局、俄罗斯联邦国家药物和GMP研究院（FSI "SID&GP"）和哥伦比亚药监局等15个国际组织或国外药品监管部门。其中发现9家制药企业存在严重缺陷，未通过国外监管/检查机构的现场检查（占比约11%）。

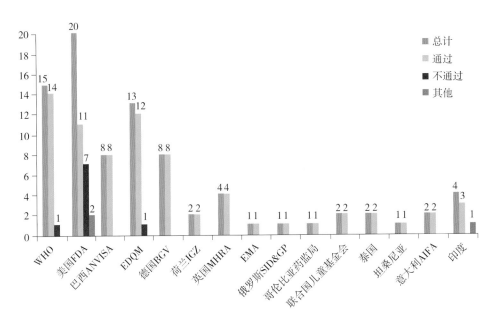

图6-2 2017年国外药品检查观察情况

与2016年相比，发现严重缺陷的企业占比基本一致（均为11%）。在9家未通过检查的企业中，多数严重缺陷项均涉及数据可靠性问题（包括重复测试至合格、删除数据、选择性使用数据、试进样、记录不及时、记录不真实、数据和记录缺失、文件记录控制不足等），部分企业涉及检验方法错误、质量管理体系存在系统性缺陷、故意隐瞒阿莫西林合成中间体等问题。总体上，数据可靠性问题较为突出，这也是2017年国内企业接受国外检查发现严重缺陷的主要方面。对于未通过检查的药品生产企业，已经要求各地加强日常监管督促企业持续合规，同时将观察检查发现的问题，作为风险信号，在下一年度跟踪检查中也一并考虑加强跟踪。

2017年检查观察共涉及170个产品，包括98个原料药、26个口服固体制剂、33个注射剂、10个生物制品、3个其他产品。在84次检查中涉及原料药的检查共46次，约占全部检查次数的55%；涉及注射剂的检查15次，占比18%；涉及口服固体制剂的检查13次，约占全部检查次数15%；涉及生物制品的检查8次，占比10%。

表6-1 不同检查机构检查药品类型分布情况

检查机构		WHO	EDQM	美国FDA	德国BGV	巴西ANVISA	其他机构	合计
药品类型	原料药	18	16	26	11	5	22	98
	口服固体制剂	2	0	6	6	1	11	26
	注射剂	6	0	9	1	4	13	33
	生物制品	5	0	0	0	1	4	10
	其他	0	1	2	0	0	0	3
	合 计	31	17	43	18	11	50	170

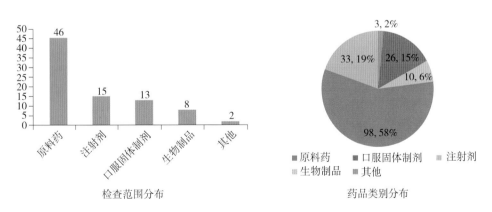

图6-3 不同剂型检查情况分布

二、发现的主要问题

（一）整体情况分析

2017年国外观察检查工作共发现缺陷项1071项，依据2010版中国GMP正文章节对缺陷项进行分类分析发现：质量控制与质量保证、文件管理、设备、厂房与设施、确认与验证、物料与产品六个类别的缺陷占了全部缺陷的88%。与2016年相比，"厂房与设施"部分缺陷由第6位上升至第4位，占比由9.1%增加至11.0%，呈现增长趋势，其余缺陷分布情况基本一致。

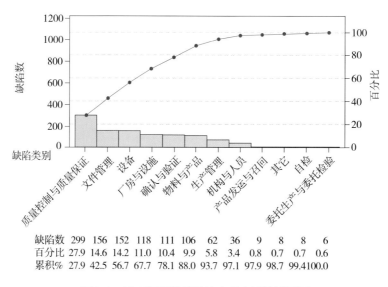

缺陷数	299	156	152	118	111	106	62	36	9	8	8	6
百分比	27.9	14.6	14.2	11.0	10.4	9.9	5.8	3.4	0.8	0.7	0.7	0.6
累积%	27.9	42.5	56.7	67.7	78.1	88.0	93.7	97.1	97.9	98.7	99.4	100.0

图6-4　2017年国外药品检查观察缺陷排列图

在国外药品GMP检查中，"质量控制与质量保证"部分共提出了299条缺陷，占总缺陷数的27.9%，位居首位，主要问题集中在偏差处理与CAPA、实验室计算机化分析仪器的管理、变更控制、产品质量回顾分析、超标/超趋势结果处理、微生物检验管理、检验相关物料管理、取样及实验室未遵循控制程序的规定。"文件管理"部分出现的缺陷居第二位，主要问题集中在记录完整性和可追溯性、文件完整性、文件的生命周期管理、记录操作四个方面。"设备"部分的缺陷居第三位，主要问题包括设备的使用与清洁、维护与维修、校准、设计选型安装改造、制水系统管理。"厂房与设施"部分的缺陷主要集中在降低污染和交叉污染的措施、厂房设施的生命周期管理、环境控制、人员进出控制。"确认与验证"方面的主要问题包括验证的科学性、验证管理、验证有效性。"物料与产品"部分出现的缺陷项集中在物料与产品标识、供应商管理、物料流程管理、放行管理、物料与产品标准的合规性等五个方面。

（二）部分国外药品监管／检查机构缺陷分布情况

尽管不同药品监管/检查机构对药品生产企业检查的重点存在一定差异，但通过对2017年国外观察检查中的缺陷情况分析发现缺陷分布情况基本一致。

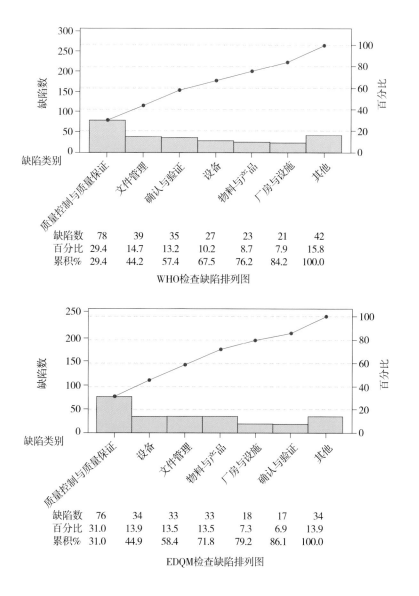

WHO检查缺陷排列图

EDQM检查缺陷排列图

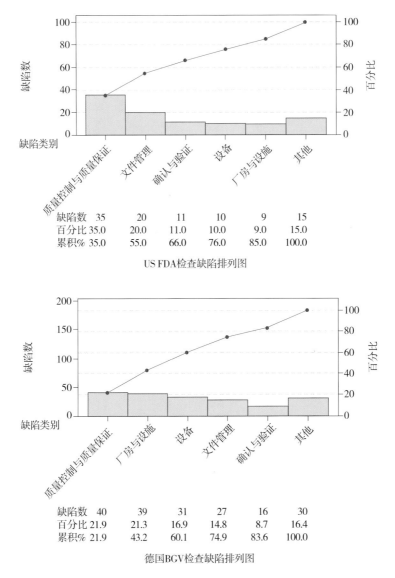

US FDA检查缺陷排列图

缺陷数	35	20	11	10	9	15
百分比	35.0	20.0	11.0	10.0	9.0	15.0
累积%	35.0	55.0	66.0	76.0	85.0	100.0

德国BGV检查缺陷排列图

缺陷数	40	39	31	27	16	30
百分比	21.9	21.3	16.9	14.8	8.7	16.4
累积%	21.9	43.2	60.1	74.9	83.6	100.0

图6-5　WHO、EDQM、US FDA 及德国BGV检查缺陷分布

　　与整体检查缺陷分布情况相同，WHO、EDQM、US FDA 及德国BGV的检查发现在质量控制与质量保证、文件管理、设备、物料与产品、确认与验证、厂房与设施等六个部分出现的缺陷相对较多。

ANNUAL REPORT OF DRUG INSPECTION 2017

Annual Inspection Report Series
of National Medical Products
Administration

Written by Center for Food and Drug

Inspection (CFDI)

Foreword

In 2017, China Food and Drug Administration (hereinafter referred to as CFDA) organized to conduct a total of 751 inspections throughout the year, including pre-approval inspection, generic drug consistency on-site inspection, pharmaceutical GMP follow-up inspection, unannounced inspection, overseas inspections for imported pharmaceuticals, GSP unannounced inspection and GMP observation inspection by foreign organizations.

Overview of Pharmaceutical Inspection Tasks in 2017

Inspections	Amount of Inspected Enterprises / Varieties	Amount of Inspectorates	Amount of Inspections
Pre-approval inspection	52	47	168
Generic drug consistency on-site inspection	12	8	38
Pharmaceutical GMP follow-up inspection	428	296	1234
Unannounced inspection for pharmaceuticals	57	55	183
Overseas inspections for imported pharmaceuticals	51	41	148
GSP unannounced inspection	67	62	202
GMP observation inspection by foreign organizations	84	84	92
Total	751	593	2065

Contents

Chapter Ⅴ   GSP inspection

Chapter Ⅵ   GMP observation inspection by foreign organizations

Chapter I
Pre-approval inspection

In 2017, CFDA carried out the pre-approval inspection and for-cause inspection according to the regulatory documents of *Provisions for Drug Registration* and *Requirements for On-site Verification for Drug Registration*, and in addition, it performed the on-site inspection of generic drug quality and efficacy consistency according to *CFDA Announcement on Matters Related to the Consistency Evaluation of the Quality and Efficacy of Generic Drugs* (2017, No. 100).

I. Basic information of inspection

There were 68 inspection tasks totally in 2017. A total of 168 person-times, 47 inspection teams have been sent out to conduct on-site inspections on 52 varieties; 45 pre-approval on-site inspection reports have been completed, of which 42 passed the inspection, accounting for 93.3%; and 3 failed, accounting for 6.7%.

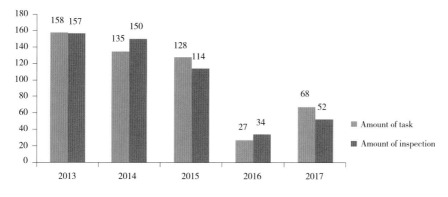

Figure 1-1   Diagram of the Number of Pre-approval Inspection Tasks in Recent Five Years

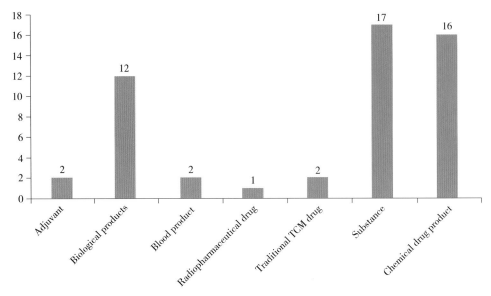

Figure 1-2   Diagram of Dosage Form Distribution in Pre-approval Inspections in 2017

II. Main findings

In the pre-approval inspections in 2017, such problems in data integrity as untraceable data and untruthful application dossier were not prominent. This is in line with the fact that most of the pre-approval inspection tasks in 2017 have been verified by clinical trial data. However, the pre-market approval GMP compliance problem is relatively common, indicating that the company's quality management system during the drug development process is relatively weak, and there is insufficient attention to the conformity of GMP. In 2017, the following problems in enterprise's development process were detected: insufficient implementation of pharmaceutical GMP and deviation and out of specification investigation insufficiency, and process validation being not scientific. The details are as follows:

(I) Insufficient implementation of pharmaceutical GMP in pilot-scale experiment or transfer process

At present, most enterprises have realized that quality management is needed during the process of transfer from R&D to production technology, but there are still deficiencies. Some enterprises still do not include this process in the GMP system of pharmaceuticals, and there are phenomena such as unclear responsibilities of personnel, insufficient understanding of production department on the variety and process knowledge, and failure of the R&D department to implement process validation to fully comply with the GMP regulations of pharmaceuticals.

(II) Insufficient investigation of deviation and out of specification results

There are cases where there are deviations and out of specification results that cannot be investigated in time, or investigations are insufficient and root causes cannot be found. In particular, when abnormal data that deviated from the trend were found in the stability test, no enough attention was paid to it, and the subsequent investigation of reasons became very difficult.

(III) Process validation is not scientific or sufficient

Some enterprises had insufficient preclinical studies on products and processes and had insufficient understanding on the process, and their design of pharmaceutical process validation protocol was unscientific. Deviations in process validation could not be recorded and analyzed in accordance with the GMP requirements of pharmaceuticals, and root causes could not be found and corrective and preventative actions could not be taken. Some enterprises even used three consecutive batches of qualified products as the criteria for the process validation.

III. On-site inspection of the consistency evaluation of quality and efficacy of generic drugs

On November 23, 2017, CFDA initiated inspections of consistency evaluation varieties for the first time of generic drugs. 7 varieties in the first time of on-site inspections were completed on the basis of the completion of the filing review. A total of six inspection teams were sent to conduct inspections on seven development and production units of seven varieties, involving nine sites. At the same time, on-site inspections were also conducted on the domestic originator of five varieties (two enterprises). Specific inspection varieties are shown in the following table:

Table 1-1   Varieties of on-site inspection of domestic originator

Serial No.	Inspection varieties	Specification	Inspecting enterprises
1	Nimodipine tablets	30mg	Bayer Pharmaceutical Health Co., Ltd.
2	Acarbose tablets	50mg; 100mg	
3	Risperidone tablets	1mg; 2mg	Xi'an Janssen Pharmaceutical Co., Ltd
4	Flunarizine hydrochloride capsules	5mg	
5	Domperidone tablets	5mg; 10mg	

Table 1-2   Varieties of on-site inspection of the consistency evaluation of generic drugs

Serial No.	Inspection varieties	Specification	Inspecting enterprises
1	Alfacalcidol tablets	0.25μg; 0.5μg	Chongqing Yaopharma Pharmaceutical Limited Liability Company

continue table

Serial No.	Inspection varieties	Specification	Inspecting enterprises
2	Amitriptyline hydrochloride tablets	25mg	Hunan Dongting Pharmaceutical Company Limited
3	Escitalopram oxalate tablets	10mg	Hunan Dongting Pharmaceutical Company Limited
4	Amoxicillin capsules	0.25g	Zhejiang Conba Bio-Pharmaceutical Co., Ltd.
5	Atorvastatin calcium tablets	10mg; 20mg	Beijing Jialin Pharmaceutical Company Limited
6	Amlodipine besylate tablet	5mg (on the basis of $C_{20}H_{25}ClN_{2O5}$)	Jiangsu Yellow River Pharmaceutical Co., Ltd.
7	Entecavir dispersible tablets	0.5mg	Jiangxi Qingfeng Pharmaceutical Co., Ltd.

Chapter II
Pharmaceutical GMP follow-up inspection

In 2017, the follow-up inspection of pharmaceutical GMP followed the principle of "risk-based and variety-focused", and adopted various methods such as "double randomization" and "lookback". Based on of the summarization of the past two years of follow-up inspection experience, a comprehensive analysis was conducted on national sampling, monitoring of adverse reactions and other risk signals to formulate national drug inspection plans, and carry out GMP follow-up inspections as planned.

I . Basic information of inspection

According to the 2017 *National Drug Inspection Plan*, 465 drug manufacturers were scheduled be subject to GMP follow-up inspections, including 315 enterprises that had high risk and 150 enterprises that had been selected into the "double randomization" plan. Among them, 37 enterprises were not qualified for the on-site inspection because they did not pass the 2010 GMP certification, the drug GMP certificate was recovered, and there was no corresponding drug approval number. Throughout the year, 428 enterprises were given drug GMP follow-up inspections (478 enterprise-times), an increase of 234% from the same period of 2016. Enterprises that did not comply with GMP have been dealt with in accordance with the law.

Table 2-1   Designation of inspectorates

Total amount of inspections (enterprises)	Amount of inspectorates	Person-time(s) of inspectors
428	296	1234

Table 2-2   Inspection distribution

Category		Amount of actual inspections enterprise - time(s)
High risk enterprises	(1) The enterprises that the conclusion of the last follow-up inspection was not passing, or showed the presence of critical defects or more than three major defects, or the warning letter was sent during the last follow-up inspection. (2) The enterprises that the pre-approval inspection found it was necessary to carry out follow-up inspections. (3) High risk defects was found by the overseas drug regulatory administration inspection. (4) The enterprises notified by CFDA to be included in the 2015 unannounced inspection	114
	Vaccine bioproduct manufacturing enterprises	39
	Blood product manufacturers	26
	In 2016, failed in the national sampling and many problems were detected during the sampling	27
	Adverse reaction monitoring found ADR or warning events	8
	Specific inspection	123
Enterprises subject to double random inspections	Narcotic drugs, psychotropic drugs and precursor pharmaceuticals manufacturing enterprises	15
	Chinese herbal medicines and herbal pieces prepared for decoction	48
	Provincial certified enterprise in 2016	30
	Herbal extract	15
	Biochemicals	17
	TCM injection	16
Total	Unit: enterprise - time(s)	478
	Unit: enterprise(s)	428

In 2017, there were 37 enterprises that did not pass the GMP inspection requirements, accounting for 8.6%, and about 108 enterprises were issued withe warning letter, accounting for 25%. Of the 37 companies that did not meet the inspection requirements. The distribution was as follows:

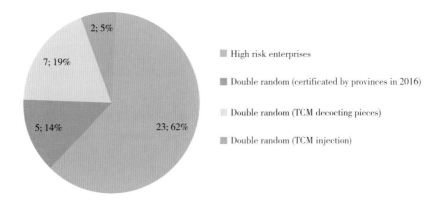

Figure 2-1   2017 Distribution of enterprises that did not meet the GMP requirements of follow-up inspections
Legend: The reasons for the non-compliance of inspections included serious violations of GMP, suspected illegal activities, and unstable product quality etc. Different handling measures could be adopted for non-compliance due to different reasons

Ⅱ. Main findings

(Ⅰ) Overall situation

The inspections on 428 drug manufacturers identified a total of 4339 defects, including 3,512 defects involving the general rule of GMP for pharmaceuticals, 224 defects involving the computer system appendices, 200 defects involving the appendices for sterile drugs, and 116 the defects involving the TCM decocting pieces.

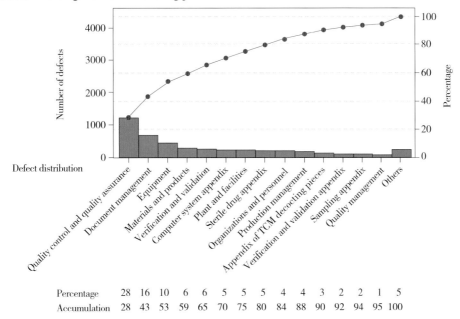

Figure 2-2   Distribution of defect items in GMP follow-up inspections

According to Figure 2-2, the defects found in the Quality Control and Quality Assurance section are the most prominent, with a total of 1,205 defects, accounting for 28%, followed by document management, accounting for 16% of the total, and then by equipment defects (ranking the third), accounting for 10%. The clauses that corresponded to non-conformity items proposed based on the defects were analyzed, and the clauses that corresponded to defects items that were submitted for more than 20 times were sorted out; they are shown below:

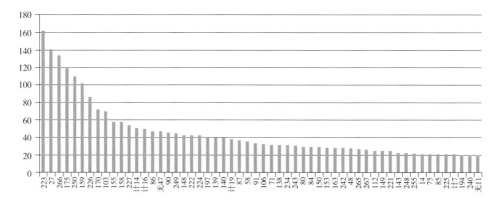

Figure 2–3　Distribution of non-conformity items detected in drug GMP follow-up inspection

Legend: "计" represents the appendix of the computer system, "无" represents the appendix of sterile drugs

The clause that corresponded to the most defects was Article 223 (Drug Testing), followed by Article 27 (Personnel Training), by Article 266 (Product Quality Review) (ranking third), by Article 175 (batch record) (ranking fourth), and by Article 250 (deviation investigation and preventive measures) (ranking fifth).

On the whole, the current defects in China's pharmaceutical manufacturing enterprises are relatively concentrated on the following items: quality control and quality assurance, document management, equipment, materials and products, qualification and validation, computer system appendix, premises and facilities, sterile drug appendix, organization and personnel, production management, appendix of TCM decocting pieces, qualification and validation appendix, sampling appendix and quality management, accounted for 95% of the total and the defects in the first eight items accounted for 80%. Some common problems included:

(1) The drug inspection procedures did not meet the requirements, some analysis methods were not verified, the management of reference products, standard substance and strains for inspection was not standardized, the relevant inspection records were not sufficiently controlled, the records were incomplete, and the traceability was poor.

(2) The training management failed to meet the requirements, the training plan and the training protocol were not well-targeted, the training effects on some personnel were poor, and

some of the work contents were not covered in the training.

(3) The product quality review regulations were unreasonable, the review did not cover all the crucial information, the review data were inconsistent, and the abnormalities found during review were not coped with corresponding measures.

(4) The batch record information was incomplete, the traceability was poor, and sometimes the recording was not standardized and untimely.

(5) The deviation management system could not operate effectively, no investigation was carried out for some deviations, and the investigations of some deviations were insufficient.

(6) There was no description on some operations in the technological procedure or the description was unclear, and for some of the information, the technological procedure was not revised in time after the change.

(7) The material management was not standardized, the relevant sign and record information were incomplete, the traceability was poor, and the storage environment failed to meet the requirements.

(8) In terms of the appendixes of the computer system, the main defects included the unreasonable permission setting, the insufficiency of electronic data management, and the incomplete audit follow-up functions.

(9) In terms of the appendix of sterile drugs, the problems concerning the culture medium simulated filling test and the monitoring of the clean area were relatively concentrated, including the unscientific operation in the medium simulated filling test as well as the failure of the clean area monitoring records to be included in the batch production records, etc.

The main problems that lead to non-conformity were analyzed through the defect analysis of the enterprise that failed to meet the requirements of inspections:

(1) There were serious data integrity problems: the detection after system time was modified, the key data were non-traceable, the original records, original maps, raw data, and computation processes were missing, the contents of original records of inspection were inconsistent, the integration parameters were maliciously modified, the maps were indiscriminately used, the production and inspection records were managed in disorder, the records were written prematurely, and no authority management and effective control were exercised on the the analytical instrument's computer system.

(2) The quality management system could not operate effectively and compromised by systemic problems. For example the qualifications and quantity of personnel did not match the production requirements, no effective identification and investigation of deviations and out of s results, deviation processing system, and change control system would be out of control.

(3) The material quality control did not meet the requirements. For example, no effective infrared identification according to the *Chinese Pharmacopoeia* (2015 edition) and

inconsistency in materials account.

(4) Excipients were added to prescriptions without the registration and approval and the production was initiated after the key process parameters were modified without authorization.

(5) The sub-packaging breached the regulations on the outsourcing of TCM decocting pieces.

(6) The product quality was not controllable.

(7) The actual production process was inconsistent with the registration application.

(Ⅱ) Inspection of vaccine biological product manufacturing enterprises

In 2017, complete-coverage inspections were conducted on vaccine manufacturers. Except for 1 enterprise that did not receive the inspections due to relocation, production suspension and planned cancellation of GMP certificates, the remaining 39 enterprises were inspected.

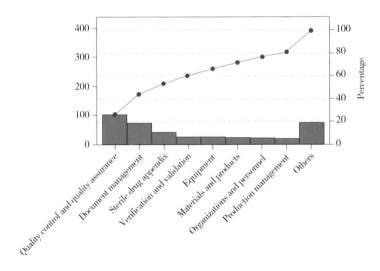

Figure 2–4　Distribution diagram of defects in vaccine manufacturers

In the defect distribution of vaccine manufacturing enterprises, the defects are mainly found on quality control and quality assurance, document management, sterile drug appendix, qualification and validation, equipment, materials and products, organization and personnel, and production management. The relatively prominent problems found during the inspection are as follows:

(1) There are certain deficiencies in the implementation of process validation, and the critical quality attributes, critical process parameters, and scope of the product were not determined.

(2) The aseptic process simulation test did not consider the worst conditions; failed to start the simulation from the first step of aseptic operation.

(3) Some enterprises used a bottle of stock solution for the preparation of multiple batches of finished products, and there were risks of contamination as the bottles were opened for several times

(4) The specifications for adjuvant could not reflect the performance of the adjuvant, and the adjuvant preparation process and performance were not verified.

(5) The uniformity validation of the preparation and subpackaging of semi-finished products had the problem of insufficient sampling.

(6) Some enterprises recruited temporary personnel to perform quality control work due to the seasonality of product production.

(7) Some enterprises failed to strictly implement the 2015 version of the Pharmacopoeia; for example, the no genome -wide sequencing was performed on the main attenuated vaccine seeds.

(8) Some enterprises did not complete annual quality review, and they did not include unqualified batches of examination, approval and issuance as well as the batches of withdrawals into statistical analysis.

(III) Inspections of blood product manufacturers

In 2017, complete-coverage inspections were conducted on blood product manufacturing enterprises. Except for one enterprise that was not subject to inspection due to the withdrawn of GMP certificates for pharmaceuticals, the remaining 26 blood product manufacturers were subject to followed up inspections.

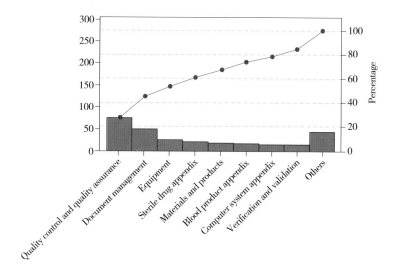

Figure 2–5   Distribution diagram of defects in blood product manufacturers

In the defect distribution of blood product manufacturing enterprises, the defects are mainly found in quality control and quality assurance, document management, equipment, sterile drug appendix, materials and products, blood product appendix, computer system appendix, and qualification and validation. The relatively prominent problems found during the inspection are as follows:

(1) For some enterprises, the aluminum ion content during the product's term of validity was on the rise, and the enterprises did not initiate relevant investigations nor carried out a thorough investigation.

(2) Some enterprises had ethanol recovery, but the related studies were deficient.

(3) The annual quality review report failed to guide subsequent improvement and upgrading.

(IV) Inspection of four categories of specific products

In accordance with the 2017 inspection plan, four categories of products, including the propyl gallate product series, citicoline sodium, vinpocetine injection, and Danshen injection, were inspected. A total of 1,243 defects were detected, among which 365 defects (including 4 critical defects, 31 major defects, and 330 general defects) were in the inspection on propyl gallate product series, 59 defects (including 6 major defects and 53 general defects) were detected in the inspection on citicoline sodium, 486 defects (including 38 major defects and 448 general defects) were detected in the injection on the Dashen injection and 333 defects (including 26 major defects and 307 general defects) were detected in the inspection on vinpocetine Injection, with the specific distribution as follows:

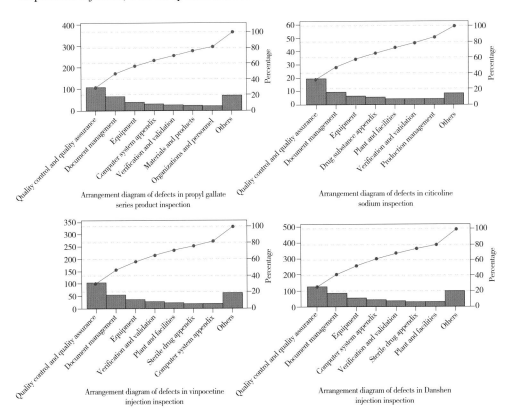

Figure 2-6   Distribution and arrangement diagram of defects in manufacturers of four categories of products

The distribution of defects in the above four categories of products was basically consistent with that of defects in the overall inspection. During the inspection process, the inspectorates selected products with higher risk for inspection based on the principle of risk according to the fact some enterprises did not manufacture the corresponding products recently. The inspections found that the problems of the enterprises in deviation handling, change control, validation scientificity, equipment maintenance, record integrity, data management standardization, annual product quality review etc. were relatively prominent. The critical defects included systematic problems in the quality management system, the conformity of quality control of critical materials with requirements, manufacturing after the unauthorized changes in prescriptions, and the presence of risks of major pollution and cross-contamination.

(V) Double random inspections

In 2017, 141 enterprises were subject to double random inspections, a total of 1283 defects were found in the inspection, including 8 critical defects, 122 major defects and 1153 general defects. The specific distribution is as follows:

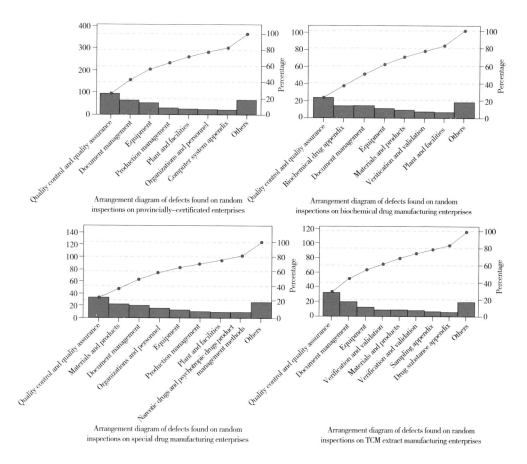

Arrangement diagram of defects found on random inspections on provincially-certificated enterprises

Arrangement diagram of defects found on random inspections on biochemical drug manufacturing enterprises

Arrangement diagram of defects found on random inspections on special drug manufacturing enterprises

Arrangement diagram of defects found on random inspections on TCM extract manufacturing enterprises

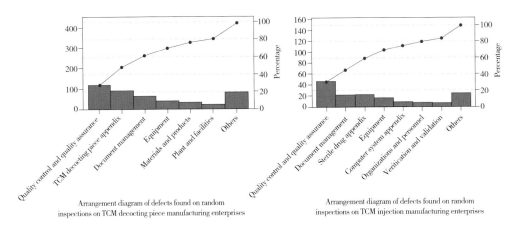

Arrangement diagram of defects found on random
inspections on TCM decocting piece manufacturing enterprises

Arrangement diagram of defects found on random
inspections on TCM injection manufacturing enterprises

Figure 2-7　Distribution and arrangement diagram of defects found in the "double random" inspections

On the whole, defects in the quality control and quality assurance parts ranked first in the inspections on manufacturing enterprises of different categories of products. According to the different types of manufacturing enterprises, there were certain differences in the defect non-conformity. The distribution of defects found in double-random inspections on provincial certification enterprises, Chinese herbal extract manufacturing enterprises, and traditional Chinese medicine injection manufacturing enterprises was basically consistent with the overall distribution of defects. In inspections of biochemical drug manufacturers, the defects of non-conformity with the requirements of the appendix of biochemical drugs ranked second, and the defects were mainly the deficiency in supply chain management and measures to avoid cross-contamination. The inspections on the manufacturing enterprises of narcotic drugs, psychotropic drugs and precursor chemicals found the non-conformity with the *Administrative Measures for the Production of Narcotic Drugs and Psychotropic Drugs*. The main problems were mainly found in the control of special drugs, including the control of the remaining samples, and the unqualified products during the production. Among the clauses that corresponded the non-conformity items found in the inspections of TCM decocting pieces, the clause that ranked No. 2 was appendix of TCM decocting pieces, and the main problems included the inspection of purchased medicinal materials, sample retention, medicinal material maintenance, personnel quality, and operational standardization.

Chapter III
Unannounced inspection for pharmaceuticals

In accordance with the *Measures for Unannounced Inspection of Drugs and Medical Device*, in 2017 the CFDA carried out unannounced inspections and relevant extended inspections on drug manufacturers.

I. Basic information of inspection

In 2017, CFDA carried out 57 drug GMP unannounced inspections. They involved 21 provinces (municipalities) including Jilin, Sichuan, and Fujian, including 5 biological product manufacturers (including blood products), 14 general chemical drug manufacturers, 28 manufacturers of TCM drug products, 7 manufacturers of TCM decocting pieces, and 3 domestic manufacturers of TCM extracts. Of the 57 unannounced inspections conducted in 2017, the manufacturers of TCM drug product accounted the highest proportion, accounting for 49% of all. TCM decocting pieces accounted for about 12%, general chemical drug products accounted for about 25%, and biological products accounted for about 9%.

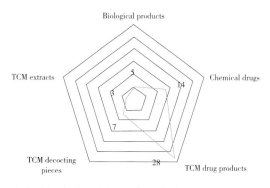

Figure 3-1   Distribution of dosage forms in drug unannounced inspections

A total of 39 companies were detected with problems in unannounced inspections throughout the year, accounting for about 68% of the total, and 27 companies that had critical defeats have been withdrawn the GMP certificates by the provincial administration or dealt with in accordance with the law.

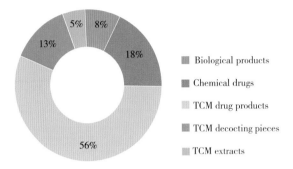

5% 8%
13%
18%
56%

- Biological products
- Chemical drugs
- TCM drug products
- TCM decocting pieces
- TCM extracts

Figure 3–2 Distribution of serious problems in drug unannounced inspections

The 2017 unannounced inspections focused more on the inspections of TCM product manufacturing enterprises, and 30 inspections involving 129 person-times were dispatched for the organization of unannounced inspections of 38 enterprises of TCM drug product, TCM decocting pieces and TCM extracts. Among them, 16 enterprises were found to have problems in the exploratory research and tests, and 12 enterprises were reported by complaint letters and visits. There were 8 enterprises that carried out extended inspections on inspection-detected problems, and 2 enterprises were subject to higher risk. The unannounced inspections on 38 TCM manufacturing enterprises, a total of 29 did not meet the relevant requirements. Among them, 21 enterprises were withdrawn GMP certificates for pharmaceuticals, 7 enterprises met the requirements, and 2 enterprises had no relevant production qualifications.

II. Main findings

(I) Major problems found in TCM product manufacturers

1. Manufacturing enterprises of Chinese patent medicines

(1) Failure to conform to the prescription standards for the feeding.

The inspections found that, the manufacturing enterprises in breach with the regulations lowered the requirement to such an extent that the final products satisfied the legal specifications without the consideration of the drug safety, effectiveness and patient's rights and interests; failed to conform to the prescription standards for the feeding deliberately. For examples:

- In Hubei kangyuan pharmaceutical co. LTD, the formula of production and feeding of a batch of deerhorn glue was the upper layer of foam when the camel skin was decocted, and then the glue obtained from the buckskin decoction, but no deerhorn was seen in the production prescriptions. The formula of production and feeding of a batch of tortoise shell glue was mainly based on a single miscellaneous skin glue and a variety of miscellaneous skin glue, then some unqualified glue was added, and finally about 5% of turtle shell glue was added.

- In Jilin xinhui pharmaceutical co. LTD, the actual feeding amount of 437 batches of Huoxiangzhengqi liquid licorice extract was only 18% of the standard feeding amount, and the actual feeding amount of patchouli oil was only 28% of the standard feeding amount.

(2) Violation of the legal preparation methods and unauthorized changes to the process.

The problems found in the unannounced inspections in 2017 were: the extraction some of Chinese crude drugs that should be extracted in the prescription failed to be based on the standards in order to reduce production costs or use unqualified raw medicinal materials; instead, direct feeding was performed after the smashing. The examples are as follows:

- The prescription of Yankening tablets consists of five medicinal materials, among which phellodendron bark needed separate decoction – water decoction for three times; after combination and concentration, ethanol was added to let them stand and filtered, and finally ethanol was recovered and concentrated. Due to the reasons for reducing the cost of raw materials and lowering the cost of process production, the phellodendron bark was directly smashed and fed into the preparation process, and the unannounced inspection found that three enterprises had the above problems.

- As for the Qingrejiedu tablets, the detection index of jasminoidin content ($\geqslant 0.6$mg/tablet) was increased in the third supplement of the *Chinese Pharmacopoeia* (2010 edition). Some enterprises failed to pass the test on cape jasmine fruit fed in the production, so in addition to normal production, each batch of product preparation process also needed the separate addition of the original powder of cape jasmine fruit to ensure that the jasminoidin content of the final product met the requirements as shown in the inspection.

(3) To cope with supervision and inspection, relevant record files were fabricated.

The unannounced inspections in 2017 found that multiple enterprises had two or even three sets of material accounts, material warehousing and ex-warehousing records, and production batch records.

- Hubei kangyuan pharmaceutical co. LTD had three sets of internal accounts, a real set for internal use for the enterprise, a second set as the "low yield" accounts set up to cope with the unqualified situation in the sampling for the expected relieve of punishment, and a third set as the "high yield" account to respond to market feedback of relatively low price.

- There were two sets of material account and batch production records in Anhui jiren pharmaceutical co. LTD , a set used to respond to supervision and inspection, with the prescription and production process completely consistent with the registration standards, and the other set as the actual batch production record, which was inconsistent with the registration standards.

2. Manufacturing enterprises of TCM decocting pieces

In 2017, the unannounced inspections on TCM decocting pieces were mainly directed to the direct subpackaging and sales of purchased TCM decocting pieces, the non-complying inspections on the purchased TCM decocting pieces or the processed products, as well as problems in dyeing and weight gain. The inspection found that in response to the supervision and inspection, some enterprises had the behaviors of fabricating batch production records and batch inspection records.

(1) Direct packaging and sales of purchased decocting pieces.

- All the decocting pieces in the finished product warehouse of TCM decocting pieces of Bozhou haomen TCM decocting pieces co. LTD had no material warehouse card. The storekeeper only set up the finished product warehousing and classification account after sales. The saffron product retention record showed that, since October 2016, the enterprise had produced 3 batches of saffron (161101, 161201, 170201), but the enterprise was unable to provide batch production records for the three batches.

- The yellow rice wine was needed by Anguo lulutong TCM decocting pieces co. LTD as a supplementary material for the production of prepared rehmannia root, solomonseal rhizome, wine-prepared desert cistanche, wine-prepared *fructus corni*, and wine-prepared glossy privet fruit. The above varieties had normal production since 2016, but the enterprise's 2017 Excipient Total Account and Classification Detail of the yellow rice wine for production used in 2017 were inconsistent with the physical presence on the site, and the enterprise failed to provide VAT invoices for sales of rice wine by the supply units.

- A TCM decocting pieces manufacturing enterprise affiliated to Wushan medical company suspended the production after the expiration date of the *Drug Production License* and transferred the plant. However, the relevant personnel of the enterprise continued the direct purchasing of TCM decocting pieces and the direct repackaging, and indiscriminately used the production batch number before the production suspension, and engaged the marketing through its superior pharmaceutical company.

(2) Failure to follow the standards for the full inspection of purchased or sold traditional Chinese medicines and TCM decocting pieces.

- Failure to provide registration records for the corresponding medicinal material testing equipment.
- Absence of references for the medicinal material testing and capillary columns for drug testing, and no detection capability for corresponding item, but a full inspection report was still issued.

(3) Batch production records were untrue.

- The use log of the main production equipment could not be provided, the used amount of the specific medicinal materials in batch production records showed a difference of 5 times from the amount used for the requisition list, and some of the batches of production adjuvants had inconsistent batch production records before and after.
- The employee's signature in the batch record was untrue.

3. Production records of TCM extracts

In 2017, two low-priced Huoxiangzhengqi liquid production enterprises were selected for unannounced inspections. At the same time, the inspections were extended to three glycyrrhiza extract and patchouli oil production factories of TCM extracts. It was found that the enterprises still had different forms of violations with the *Notice of the CFDA on Strengthening the Supervision and Administration of Extraction and Extracts in the Production of Traditional Chinese Medicines* (SYJYHJ (2014) No. 135). The specific problems are as follows:

- On January 26, 2016, Sichuan hebang xudong pharmaceutical co. LTD filed the glycyrrhiza extract and patchouli oil for recording according to the regulations. At the same time, since February 2016, it began to conduct the extraction of glycyrrhiza extract and patchouli oil privately. The enterprise also maliciously fabricated the bills of the relevant Chinese medicine extract manufacturing enterprises, and privately made the special seals of the ex-warehousing of Chinese medicine extract manufacturing companies, and made up the relevant material account and batch production records to cope with supervision and inspection.
- Guangzhou tongde pharmaceutical co. LTD, although recorded by provincial department, it had no main production device for the manufacturing of patchouli oil; instead, it purchased crude liquid from the medicinal material production base and added a refining process to the unqualified patchouli oil to obtain the product after the refining by its TCM extraction workshop and then market the final products.

(Ⅱ) Major problems found in chemical manufacturers

In 2017, a total of 14 general chemical manufacturers were subject to unannounced inspections and it turned out that 7 of them had problems. The main problems were mainly found in the following aspects.

1. The production violated the registered and approved process

Illegal purchasing of crude raw materials for the production of drug substance of the company. The enterprise could not provide the records on the source of the starting materials used to trace the production of drug substance, and could not provide relevant records used to trace the drug production and quality management process. The drug substance was released and sold without any recording on materials, production, and inspection, and key personnel failed to perform their duties.

2. The original data of inspection could not be traced and the data integrity was compromised

Open and delete the audit trail logs at will. The computer system time used by the device could be modified, and records of the system time modified in 2016 and 2017 appeared in the system log; modification in the system time could be found in the related substance detection mapping material detection maps.

Some of the out of specification investigation and treatment measures were not thorough. For example, although no abnormality was mentioned when the out of specification result investigation described the inspection and sampling process, the release could be done only after the qualification by re-sampling and reinspection.

3. Drug production using unqualified raw materials

Buying and using drug substances that were not in conformity with the 2015 edition of the Chinese Pharmacopoeia for the production and marketing of tablets; counterfeiting and changing of the label of drug substance manufacturing enterprise, and counterfeiting the inspection report of drug substance manufacturing enterprises; changing the inspection samples and retained samples, and the in-coming inspection results of some drug substances being not true; the key management personnel of the enterprise could not perform their duties according to regulations, and were directly involved in the implementation of illegal activities.

(III) Major problems found in biological product manufacturers

In 2017, a total of 5 biological product manufacturers were subject to unannounced inspection and it turned out that three of them had problems. The main problems were mainly found in the following aspects.

1. Process control data or product result data is not true

As for the 9 batches of Human Albumin used by Guangzhou danxia biopharmaceutical co. LTD to declare production and registration, the 3-month and 6-month long-term stability and

6-month acceleration test showed that, most of the actual aluminum ion detection results were higher than the 200 μg /L, a criterion specified in the Chinese Pharmacopoeia. The continuous stability investigation after the marketing of this biological product showed that, the aluminum ion detection results were inconsistent with the report, the actual inspection results did not meet the standards, and problems such as modification of sample name, deletion of detection records and re-detection were found in the enterprise.

Hangzhou puji pharmaceutical technology development co. LTD forged intermediate product and finished product test data, plasma microbial limit detection data for pig whole blood separation, pig blood refrigerated van transport temperature record, purified water system validation microbiological limit test data, cultivation room temperature monitoring data of culture medium simulated filling test, air monitoring data of clean area, the freeze-drying process batch production records of marketing batches, etc., and concealed the relevant data of the real cause for the unqualified products and falsified the time of the QC laboratory computer system.

2. The actual production process and the product registration process were inconsistent

The behavior of repeated activation operation in the catalyst activation working procedure of the actual production process of the product was inconsistent with the registered and approved process.

3. The use of raw materials, intermediates and semi-finished products that did not meet quality standards for feeding

The use of microbiologically unqualified plasma for trial batch feeding and production; the use of intermediates unqualified in the ethanol residues, bacterial endotoxins, coagulation activity, microbial limits, purity and barium chloride residues as well as semi-finished products unqualified in pH value, protein concentration and enzyme activity failure for the feeding.

4. No relevant research was conducted in the production process and batch changes

In the catalyst purification process, the ultrafiltration membrane with a molecular weight of 6000 was changed into the ultrafiltration membrane package with a molecular weight of 10,000, and no validation data supported this change; the ultrafiltration was repeated in the ultrafiltration process of the catalyst and no relevant validation studies were performed; in the main gel purification and refining working procedure, the filter element was changed, the filter element was changed to the filter cake, the material of the sterilization and filtration working procedure was changed from PVDF to PES, and no relevant validation research was conducted or the validation data were insufficient; the batch volume of the solution was changed from 20,000 to 40,000 bottles, and no relevant validation research was conducted.

5. Problems in aluminum adjuvant quality control

Not test the effect of aluminum hydroxide adjuvant on antigen adsorption, and did not study the effect of aluminum hydroxide adjuvant on product quality. Aluminum hydroxide, as the most important excipient (adjuvant), was not subject to effective quality control.

Chapter IV
Overseas inspections for imported pharmaceuticals

I. Basic information of inspection

In 2017, a total of 148 inspectors from 41 inspectorates were dispatched to complete overseas inspections for 51 categories of imported pharmaceuticals.

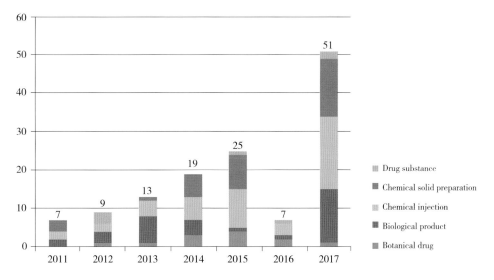

Figure 4-1　Overseas inspection tasks from 2011 to 2017

In 2017, there were many types of dosage forms for overseas inspections; in addition, the efforts of extended examinations on chemical drug products were intensified. The annual tasks covered 36 chemical products, including injections, solid drug products, and powder aerosols, etc; 14 vaccines, blood products, and therapeutic biological products; and 1 botanical drugs.

The overseas inspection tasks in 2017 covered the products at the declaration production, re-registration, supplementary application phases, and those which are normally imported and sold. The inspections were mainly concentrated in Europe and North America, and the number of inspections in India and Thailand etc. showed an increasing trend.

II. Main findings

Of the 51 varieties that were subject to on-site inspections on overseas production, 9 failed to pass inspections. According to the different stages of the product (pre-market review or post-market), they have been processed separately.Of the 8 varieties that have not been inspected on-site, the enterprises of 6 varieties took the initiative to take risk-control measures, and the rest are included in the inspection plan of next year.

A total of 665 defects were found on the site, including 27 critical defects and 140 major defects. The problems were mainly found in quality control and quality assurance, document management, and sterile drug management. Critical defects mainly included inconsistent production process, no timely reporting of major changes to Chinese organizations, the problem with the authenticity of the registration application materials, production plant facilities, equipment and production operation practices failing to effectively reduce the risk of product contamination or mixing, and the failure of exercising effective control on unqualified products.

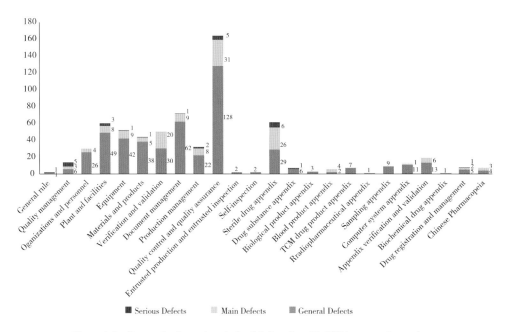

Figure 4–2　Summarization and analysis of defects found in 2017 overseas inspections

According to the statistics of the defect frequency, the defects in the part of quality control and quality assurance were the most, with a total of 164 items (24.7%), followed by those in the document management part, with a total of 72 items (accounting for 10.8%), and 61 items were found in the part of sterile drug appendix (accounting for 9.2%). Common problems included:

(1) The deviation management system could not operate effectively, no investigation was carried out for some deviations, and the investigations of some deviations were insufficient.

(2) The sampling operation and records of the drug testing did not meet the requirements; the data of the purified water production process were not monitored and validated; the testing data and environmental monitoring data were not conductive to the data saving of trend analysis methods.

(3) The information in the batch records are not sufficient, such as the amount and whereabouts of the remaining sterilized rubber plugs and aluminum caps after filling were recorded.

(4) The annual retrospective report was incomplete; for example, there was no regulation on deviation-correcting line and the warning line for the corrective analysis.

(5) The content of the technological procedure of the production was not complete, such as: lack of some of the process parameters (emulsification temperature, shear speed, etc., the longest time limit for tunnel sterilization oven, nitrogen pressure, etc.).

(6) The problems of non-scientific validation of medium simulated filling in the sterile drug appendix were more prominent, such as unreasonable validation frequency, the worst condition not including the maximum allowable number of people in production lines, and storage time after tank sterilization.

In the overseas inspection in 2017, the major problems that prevented the enterprises from passing the inspection included:

(1) Actual production process, production sites, inspection items, etc. were inconsistent with the registration and application, or major changes were implemented without being reported to Chinese organizations. For example, during the preparation of injection oil phase, the actual filtration method and filter materials were inconsistent with the registered and declared materials; the products released and exported to China were not tested in terms of the related substance test and content uniformity according to the import registration standards; the process prescriptions were changed; the actual production plants and the production address were inconsistent with the manufacturing factory and production address labeled on the imported drug registration certificate.

(2) Presence of serious problems in data reliability. For example, in multiple batches of release detection maps, the materials copied and forged using the information strips at different speeds and at different times served as materials submitted for registration and review; on-

site inspections could not provide original inspection records; the pilot batch numbers of the prescription-screened samples were inconsistent with those of relevant intermediate products and finished product inspection, and there was an inconsistency in the pilot preparation records, particle assay, releasing rate determination (finished product), and assay (naked tablet) of the same batch of samples.

(3) The production plant facilities, equipment and production operation practices failed effectively reduce the risk of product contamination or mixing. For example, the filling production line set for the hydro-acupuncture therapy was located at the same workshop for the powder injection production line (the production line had hormone products), they also shared the same air purification system, the enterprise did not conduct risk assessments nor took effective protective measures to avoid the contamination of hormonal products on other products. Filling operators needed to manually press the rubber plug into the aluminum cover, and then place it in the corresponding cavity of the filled triple-chamber bag. There were many places of sewage and garbage in the factory area. Insufficient measures were taken to prevent mosquitoes in the general production area and the factory was annually under a high temperature (up to 45 °C), without cooling measures adopted, and the doors and windows could not be closed. The screen windows were damaged in many places, and many mosquitoes and insects were found on the production site. The feeding took place under the conditions of exposure or the materials were transferred, and there was no local protection.

(4) The product quality was not controllable. For example, an on-site inspection was initiated because the import test of bacterial endotoxin project item found an unqualified result, the enterprise performed a re-determination on the item and did not meet the requirements, but still no investigation was carried out on the out-of-limit results, and no risk evaluation was performed on the product-related batches of the products and the used drug substance; the failure to perform full inspection according to the Chinese Pharmacopoeia.

Chapter V
GSP inspection

In order to further strengthen the quality supervision of drug circulation links and standardize the order of the pharmaceutical market, CFDA organized follow-up inspections of drug wholesalers and inspections on retail pharmacies.

I. Basic information of inspection

(I) Overview

In accordance with the *2017 Drug GSP Follow-up Inspection Plan*, CFDA organized follow-up inspections on a total of 55 drug wholesalers throughout the year, covering 20 provinces (autonomous regions and municipalities) including Guangdong, Sichuan and Hubei. In order to carry out the Centralized Rectification of the Drug Quality and Safety of Drugs in Pharmacies and Clinics in Urban-Rural Interfaces and in Rural Areas, CFDA also organized unannounced inspections on 12 retailing pharmacies in Liaoning, Hunan and Guizhou provinces. Compared with the 2016 inspection tasks, the inspection tasks this year increased by 34%. The inspection details were as follows:

Table 5-1　Number of tasks of GSP unannounced inspections in 2016 and 2017

Year	Number of inspected enterprises	Number of dispatches inspectors (man-time)
2016	50	77
2017	67	202
Total	117	206

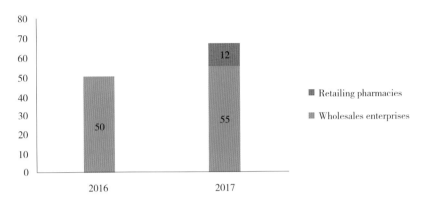

Figure 5–1   Number of tasks of GSP unannounced inspections in 2016 and 2017

(Ⅱ) Inspection principles and inspection scope

In accordance with the principle of risk management and control, the drug wholesales enterprises which provided varieties of high safety risks, had high requirements for variety storage conditions, had unqualified results in national drug sampling, and were complained of and reported, were selected for the drug GSP follow-up inspections; the "double-random" approaches were adopted in the inspection, and 55 wholesales enterprises of different types were randomly selected from national drug wholesales enterprises, and 12 retailing pharmacies were selected among the pharmacies in urban-rural interfaces and in rural areas for inspections. See the following table:

Table 5-2   Inspection scope of drug GSP

Category	Number of enterprises
Operation of narcotic drugs and psychoactive drugs (including compound preparations)	15
Business scope included biological products and cold-chain drugs	15
Newly-established enterprises	15
Unqualified national drug sampling	5
complained of and reported	5
Retailing pharmacies in urban-rural interfaces and in rural areas	12
Total	67

(Ⅲ) Inspection results

According to the Guiding Principles for On-site Inspection of Good Supply Practice, 29 operating enterprises severely violated the Good Supply Practice, and the results were judged as not passing the inspection.

(1) Wholesale enterprises engaged in the operation of narcotic drugs and psychoactive drugs (including compound preparations): 3 failed to pass the inspections, accounting for 20% of the 15 enterprises inspected.

(2) The scope included the wholesales enterprises selling biological products and cold-chain medicines: 1 company was in the state of business suspension, no conclusion was drawn from the inspection, and 6 failed to pass the inspections, accounting for 40% of the 15 enterprises inspected.

(3) Newly-established wholesales enterprises: 5 failed to pass the inspections, accounting for 33.3% of the 15 enterprises inspected.

(4) Wholesales enterprises unqualified in the national drug sampling: 2 failed to pass the inspections, accounting for 40% of the 5 enterprises inspected.

(5) Wholesales enterprises that were complained of and reported: 3 (of which 1 was within GSP certification publicity period) failed to pass the inspection, accounting for 60% of the 5 enterprises inspected.

(6) Retailing pharmacies in urban-rural interfaces and in rural areas: 10 failed to pass the inspections, accounting for 83.3% of the 12 enterprises inspected.

In summary, 19 drug wholesales enterprises failed to pass the follow-up inspection, and the rate of failure was 34.5%. 10 enterprises failed to pass the unannounced inspection of retailing pharmacies in urban-rural interfaces and in rural areas, and the rate of failure was 83.3%. Compared with the inspections in 2016, the failure rate of wholesales companies dropped significantly. Enterprises that fail to pass the inspection have been dealt with in accordance with the law.

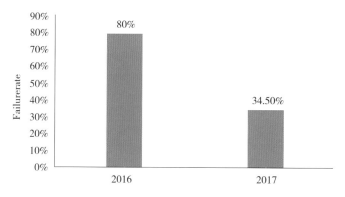

Figure 5–2   Failure rate of inspections of drug wholesales enterprises in 2016 and 2017

II. Main findings

(I) Inspections on drug wholesales company

A total of 436 defects were found in the inspection on the drug wholesales enterprises throughout the year, including 58 critical defects, 330 major defects and 48 general defects. The distribution of various types of defects is shown below.

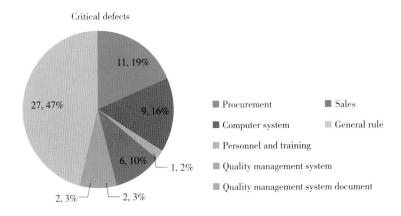

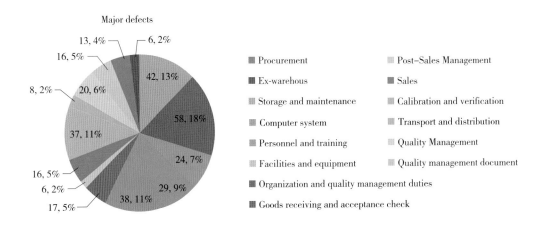

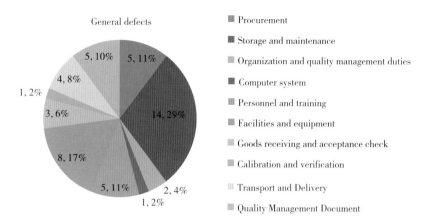

Figure 5–3 Distribution of critical defects in drug wholesales enterprises

The critical defects in drug wholesales enterprises were mainly distributed in the general rule, procurement, computer system, and sales etc. The major defects of drug wholesales enterprises were mainly in the aspects of organization and quality management responsibilities, storage and maintenance, facilities and equipment, calibration and validation. The general defects of drug wholesales enterprises were mainly distributed in storage and maintenance, facilities and equipment, procurement, personnel and training.

1. Inspections on wholesale enterprises engaged in the operation of narcotic drugs and psychoactive drugs (including compound preparations)

15 enterprises in this category had a total of 115 defects, including 10 critical defects, distributed in the general rule, computer systems, and quality management system, which accounted for 8.7% of all defects, with 90 major defects and 15 general defects.

The defects found in inspections on this type of enterprises were more often found in the aspects of organization and quality management responsibilities, calibration and validation, facilities and equipment, procurement, computer systems, personnel and training. During the on-site inspections, the inspectorates conducted targeted inspections on the conformity of operating enterprises with GSP, targeted inspections were performed on the operation of drugs subject to special management and even extended inspections were conducted on the downstream. Inspections found that most enterprises did well in the operation of special drugs and no abuse occurred. However, there were still some problems, such as: no handling of mailing certificates before the mailing of narcotic drugs and psychotropic drugs; failure to provide transportation certificates for special drugs and so on.

2. Inspections of wholesales enterprises with a business scope including biological products and cold-chain drugs

15 enterprises in this category had a total of 115 defects, including 14 critical defects, distributed in the general rule, computer systems, and procurement, which accounted for 12.2% of all defects, with 94 major defects and 7 general defects.

The defects found in inspections on this type of enterprises were more often found in the aspects of organization and quality management responsibilities, facilities and equipment, calibration and validation, storage and maintenance, computer systems, personnel and training. As such companies are engaged in the sales of refrigerated and frozen pharmaceuticals, the inspectorates paid special attention to their cold chain conditions. The common problems of enterprises are as follows: Cold storage facilities and equipment did not meet requirements; the validation was not in conformity with the regulations; the operation training for cold storage of pharmaceuticals and transportation personnel was insufficient; some temperature and humidity records were missing; after the temperature and humidity of the cold storage were out of limit, alarms and short messages could not be promptly sent; the temperature data of refrigerated drugs could not be recorded.

3. Inspections on the newly established drug wholesales enterprises

15 enterprises in this category had a total of 132 defects, including 21 critical defects, distributed in the general rule, procurement, and sales which accounted for 15.9% of all defects, with 95 major defects and 16 general defects.

The defects found in inspections on such enterprises were more often found in storage and maintenance, facilities and equipment, organization and quality management responsibilities, personnel and training, and procurement. There were more problems in the newly established enterprises than in the former two types of enterprises. The proportion of critical defects was on the rise. There were serious problems in some enterprises. For example, there were 30 defects in Shenze county pharmaceutical company yongji wholesale department, including 9 critical defects, which violated A*nnouncement of CFDA on Remediating Illegal Distribution Behaviors in Drug Circulation Field* (2016 No.94) No.1~10; Chongqing enkang medicine co. LTD had 9 defects, including 4 critical defects, which violated No. 94 Notice No. 1, No. 4, No. 5 and No. 10 items. The newly established wholesales companies had the following common problems: they failed to store the drugs according to the temperature requirements of the packaging; they failed to effectively monitor and control the temperature and humidity of the warehouse; the stacking did not meet the requirements; the pharmaceuticals and non-pharmaceuticals were not stored separately; the temperature and humidity monitoring data could not be reasonably backed up; quality management personnel was part-time or not in post.

4. Inspections of wholesales enterprises unqualified in the national drug sampling

5 enterprises in this category had a total of 36 defects, including 4 critical defects, distributed in the general rule, procurement and computer systems, which accounted for 11.1% of all defects, with 29 major defects and 3 general defects.

The defects found in inspections on this type of enterprises were more often found in the aspects of organization and quality management responsibilities, storage and maintenance, and facilities and equipment. There were common problems in the enterprise as follows: no job responsibilities established for the position; the contents of the drug quality file were incomplete; the quality management department failed to perform inspection and management sufficiently; some positions were not assigned with permission to operate on the computer system; different drug were mixed and stacked; the temperature and humidity record backup did not meet the requirements; the temperature and humidity monitoring facilities and equipment did not meet the specification requirements.

5. Inspections on the drug wholesales enterprises complained of and reported

5 enterprises in this category had a total of 38 defects, including 9 critical defects distributed in the general rule, quality management system file, computer system and sales, which accounted for 23.7% of all defects, with 22 major defects and 7 general defects.

The defects found in inspections on such enterprises were more often found in storage and maintenance, general rule, organization and quality management responsibilities. The critical defects of such enterprises were higher than those of other enterprises, and they mainly existed in the general part. The common problems in the enterprises were as follows: suspected illegal business practices; falsification and cheating; drug flow, temperature and humidity monitoring data and computer system data could not be traced; failure to store drugs at the required temperature; no effective monitoring of temperature and humidity; presence of external personnel for part-time work; quality responsible person did not perform their duties independently.

（Ⅱ）Inspections on retailing pharmacies in urban-rural interfaces and in rural areas

12 enterprises in this category had a total of 91 defects, including 31 critical defects, distributed in the general rule, procurement and acceptance check, and sales which accounted for 34.1% of all defects, with 50 major defects and 10 general defects.

The defects found by inspections on such companies were more often found in display and storage, procurement and acceptance check, and general rules. The failure rate of passing the inspections of the retailing pharmacies in urban-rural interfaces and in rural areas was 83.3%, and the proportion of critical defects was the highest. There were common problems in the enterprise as follows: Failed to provide the accompanying documents and invoices of the purchased drugs, so the source of the drug could not be traced; there were no labeled production enterprises, no outer package, no place of production or production lot number of the TCM decocting pieces; over-range marketing of drugs, and alleged purchasing of drugs from illegal channels; there was no partitioned display between the prescription drugs and over-the-counter drugs, and prescription drugs were sold on shelves; illegal sales of mifepristone tablets; prescriptions were faked and computer systems automatically generated prescriptions.

In summary, since the announcement of 2016 No.94, drug regulatory authorities at all levels conducted multiple rounds of unannounced inspections and follow-up inspections (unannounced forms) on drug distribution companies to strictly crack down on illegal activities and violations in the circulation field, and the situation of pharmaceutical operations was significantly improving. In 2016, CFDA carried out unannounced inspection on 50 drug wholesales enterprises, of which 38 had critical defects and the inspection pass rate was only 24%. This year, 55 wholesales enterprises were inspected, of which 19 had critical defects, and the inspection pass rate was 65.5%, and the business practices of the enterprises were increasingly standardized. As inspections continue to scale up, awareness of compliance in the pharmaceutical circulation industry was gradually increasing, and illegal violations were gradually reduced. The inspections have promoted virtuous competition and healthy and orderly development in the industry, providing strong guarantees for people's medication safety.

Chapter VI
GMP observation inspection by foreign organizations

According to notifications from foreign drug regulatory and inspection agencies, CFDA observed the on-site inspections on the drug manufacturing enterprises in China performed by foreign drug regulatory agencies to grasp the product export and production quality management of pharmaceutical production enterprises in China, grasp the inspections by major international organizations and foreign drug regulatory agencies, assess and analyze risk signals, and provide reference for drug inspections.

I. Basic information of inspection

The CFDA organized a total of 84 foreign observations and inspections in 2017, involving 81 enterprises, covering 23 provinces (cities or autonomous regious) including Zhejiang and Guangdong etc, of which Zhejiang, Guangdong, Beijing, Hebei, Jiangsu, and Shandong accounted for 60% of the total, which was basically the same with last year.

Inspection agencies involved in 2017 inspections and observations included 15 international organizations or foreign drug regulatory agencies such as the US Food and Drug Administration (US FDA), the World Health Organization (WHO), the European Directorate for the Quality of. Medicines & HealthCare (EDQM), the Behörde für Gesundheit und Verbraucherschutz (BGV), Brazilian Health Regulatory Agency (Anvisa), Indian Central Drugs Standard Control Organization (CDSCO), British Medicines and Health Products Administration (MHRA), Italian Medicines Agency (AIFA), Thai Food and Drug Administration, Dutch Health Care Inspectorate (IGZ), United Nations Children's Fund (UNICEF), European Medicines Agency (EMA), Tanzania Food and Drug Administration, Russian State Institute of Drugs and Good Practices (FSI "SID & GP") and Colombia Food and Drug Administration. Among them, 9 pharmaceutical companies were found to have critical defects and did not pass the on-site inspections by foreign regulatory/inspection agencies (accounting for about 11%).

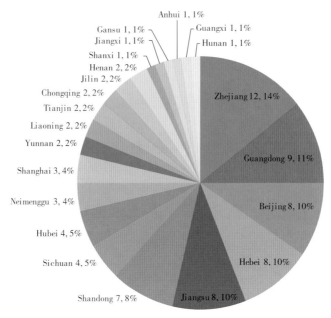

Figure 6-1   Distribution of foreign drug inspections in various provinces (cities) in 2017

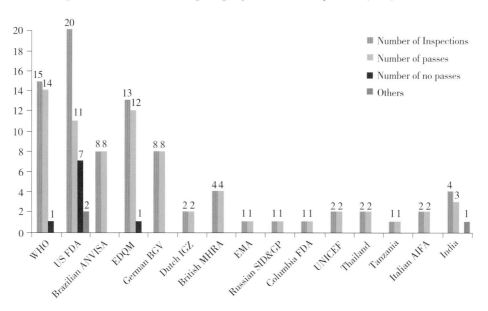

Figure 6-2   Distribution of foreign drug inspections in 2017

Compared with 2016, the overall failure rate was similar (11%). Of the nine companies that failed to pass the inspections, most of the critical defects were related to data integrity issues (including repeated testing until the qualified results were obtained, data deletion, selective use of data, test sample injection, failing to record timely, untruthful records, loss of data and records, insufficient file record control, etc.), some enterprises involved the problems of incorrect inspection methods, systematic defects in the quality management system, intentional concealment of intermediates for the synthesis of amoxicillin, etc. In general, the data integrity problem was more prominent, which was also the main reason for the increase in the failure rate of domestic enterprises to pass foreign inspections in 2017. For enterprises that have not passed inspections, local governments have been required to strengthen daily supervision and supervise the company's continuous compliance. At the same time, as a risk signal, problems discovered during observation and inspection are also considered for follow-up inspection in the next year.

The inspections and observations in 2017 involved a total of 170 products, including 98 drug substances, 26 oral solid preparations, 33 injections, 10 biological products, and 3 other products. In 84 inspections, 46 of them involved drug substance, accounting for about 55% of the total number of inspections; 15 involved injections, accounting for 18%; 13 involved oral solid preparations, accounting for about 15%; 8 involved biological products, accounting for 10%.

Table 6-1   Distribution of drug types inspected by different inspection agencies

Inspection agencies		WHO	EDQM	US FDA	German BGV	Brazilian ANVISA	Other organizations	Total
Drug types	Drug substance	18	16	26	11	5	22	98
	Oral solid preparations	2	0	6	6	1	11	26
	Injection	6	0	9	1	4	13	33
	Biological products	5	0	0	0	1	4	10
	Others	0	1	2	0	0	0	3
	Total	31	17	43	18	11	50	170

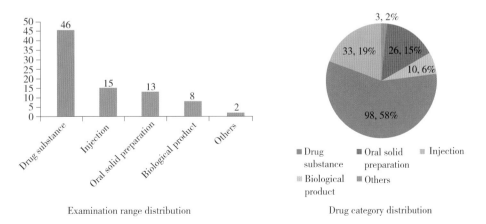

Examination range distribution   Drug category distribution

Figure 6-3   Distribution of different dosage forms

II. Main findings

(I) Analysis on overall situation

1071 defects were found in the foreign observation and inspection in 2017, and the analysis on the defect items according to the main body of 2010 version of China GMP: the defects in six categories of quality control and quality assurance, document management, equipment, premises and facilities, qualification and validation and materials and products accounted for 88% of all. Compared with 2016, the rank of the defects in the part of "premises and facilities" increased from No. 6 to No. 4, the proportion increased from 9.1% to 11.0%, showing a growing trend, and the distribution of other defects was basically the same.

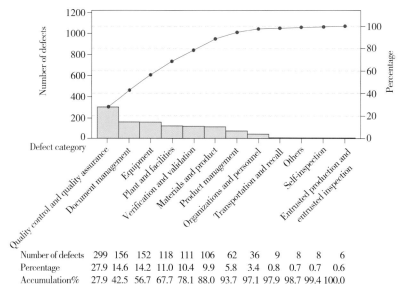

Number of defects	299	156	152	118	111	106	62	36	9	8	8	6
Percentage	27.9	14.6	14.2	11.0	10.4	9.9	5.8	3.4	0.8	0.7	0.7	0.6
Accumulation%	27.9	42.5	56.7	67.7	78.1	88.0	93.7	97.1	97.9	98.7	99.4	100.0

Figure 6-4　Arrangement diagram of defects found in foreign drug inspections and observations in 2017

In foreign drug GMP inspections, the defects in the part of "Quality Control and Quality Assurance" accounted for 27.9% of the total number of defects, which ranked first. A total of 299 defects were proposed. The main problems were mainly found on deviation handing and CAPA, management of computerized analytical instrument of laboratories, change control, product quality review, out of specification/out of trend results handing, microbiological test management, test-related material management, sampling, and non-compliance of laboratory with the control procedures. The defects found in the part of "document management" ranked the second, the main problems were found in the four aspects: record integrity and traceability, document integrity, file life cycle management, and record operation. The defects in the part of "equipment" ranked the third, and the main problems involved the use and cleaning of equipment, maintenance and repair, calibration, design and pattern selection, installation and modification, and water production system management. The defects in the part of "premises and facilities" were mainly found on measures to reduce contamination and cross-contamination, life cycle management of plant facilities, environmental control, and personnel access control. The main issues in the part of "qualification and validation" included validation scientificality, validation management, and validation effectiveness. The defects in the part of "materials and products" were mainly found on five aspects: material and product identification, supplier management, material procedure management, release management, and compliance of materials and product standards.

(II) Distribution of defects in some foreign drug regulatory/inspection agencies

Although there were certain differences in the focus of inspections by drug regulatory/inspection agencies on pharmaceutical manufacturing enterprises , the distribution of defects was basically consistent with the analysis of defects observed in foreign inspections in 2017.

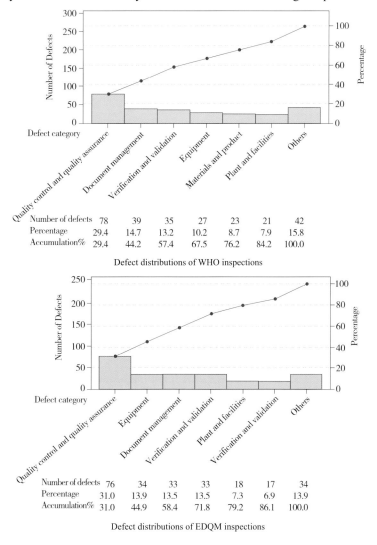

Number of defects	78	39	35	27	23	21	42
Percentage	29.4	14.7	13.2	10.2	8.7	7.9	15.8
Accumulation%	29.4	44.2	57.4	67.5	76.2	84.2	100.0

Defect distributions of WHO inspections

Number of defects	76	34	33	33	18	17	34
Percentage	31.0	13.9	13.5	13.5	7.3	6.9	13.9
Accumulation%	31.0	44.9	58.4	71.8	79.2	86.1	100.0

Defect distributions of EDQM inspections

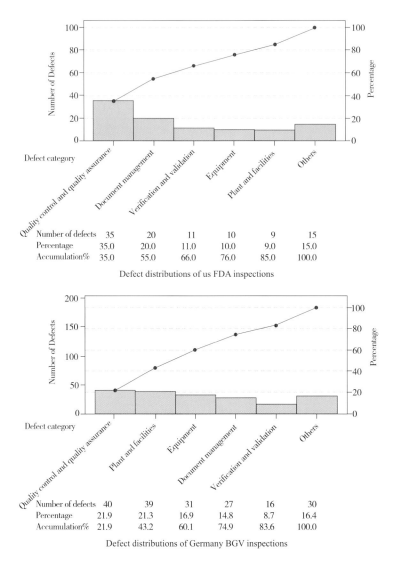

Defect category	Number of defects	Percentage	Accumulation%
Quality control and quality assurance	35	35.0	35.0
Document management	20	20.0	55.0
Verification and validation	11	11.0	66.0
Equipment	10	10.0	76.0
Plant and facilities	9	9.0	85.0
Others	15	15.0	100.0

Defect distributions of us FDA inspections

Defect category	Number of defects	Percentage	Accumulation%
Quality control and quality assurance	40	21.9	21.9
Plant and facilities	39	21.3	43.2
Equipment	31	16.9	60.1
Document management	27	14.8	74.9
Verification and validation	16	8.7	83.6
Others	30	16.4	100.0

Defect distributions of Germany BGV inspections

Figure 6–5   Defect distributions of WHO, EDQM, US FDA, and Germany BGV inspections

Similar to the overall inspection defect distribution, the number of the defects found by WHO, EDQM, US FDA and Germany BGV in six parts: quality control and quality assurance, document management, equipment, materials and products, qualification and validation, and premises and facilities, were relatively high.

(Note: The English version of this report is for reference only)